EXPERT PRACTICE

A Critical Discourse

EXPERT PRACTICE

A Critical Discourse

Alison Ferguson, Ph.D.

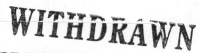
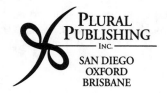

PLURAL
PUBLISHING
INC.

SAN DIEGO
OXFORD
BRISBANE

MW

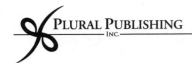

5521 Ruffin Road
San Diego, CA 92123

e-mail: info@pluralpublishing.com
Web site: http://www.pluralpublishing.com

49 Bath Street
Abingdon, Oxfordshire OX14 1EA
United Kingdom

Typeset in 10½/13 Palatino by Flanagan's Publishing Services, Inc.
Printed in the United States of America by McNaughton and Gunn

*Every attempt has been made to contact the copyright holders for material originally
printed in another source. If any have been inadvertently overlooked, the publishers will
gladly make the necessary arrangements at the first opportunity.*

Library of Congress Cataloging-in-Publication Data:

Ferguson, Alison.
   Expert practice : a critical discourse / Alison Ferguson.
        p. ; cm.
   Includes bibliographical references and index.
   ISBN-13: 978-1-59756-064-1 (pbk.)
   ISBN-10: 1-59756-064-2 (pbk.)
  1. Speech therapy. 2. Critical discourse analysis. I. Title.
   [DNLM: 1. Speech-Language Pathology—methods. 2. Communication.
3. Interprofessional Relations. 4. Linguistics. WL 340.2 F352e 2007]
   RC423.F42 2007
   616.85'506—dc22

                                                              2007025012

2/7/08

Contents

Preface

This book integrates three notions that are important to practicing speech-language pathologists: the notion of *expert*, the notion of a *critical* perspective, and the approach of *critical discourse analysis*.

Expert practice is distinguished from that of the novice through the seamless integration of past learning (both theoretical and experiential) with fast, flexible, and ethical problem-solving in response to individual cases and situations. For example, experts have been found to recognize and analyze problems through holistic pattern recognition, in contrast with the more atomistic and stepwise problem-solving of novices. This book presents the argument that the achievement of expertise brings with it an intrinsic paradox in that expert practice also demands critical reflection on practice in order to develop further—that is, the more automatic and patterned practice becomes, the more crucial it becomes to deconstruct these patterned practices in order to allow for objective examination. Without critical reflection, expert practitioners run the risk of fossilization of the very patterns that defined their expertise.

The notion of a critical perspective is part of a wider theoretical paradigm that emerged during the latter half of the twentieth century, in which a range of disciplines have drawn on the philosophical works of such scholars as Habermas and Foucault. Different disciplines and researchers who use this approach have very different agendas and methodologies, but broadly speaking, the common threads are, first, an explicit stance in which truths or facts within a discipline are seen in relation to the social and cultural context in which they emerge and operate; second, a theoretical presumption of the pivotal role of social power and its distribution in defining accepted truths; and third, an explicit agenda that the outcome of such research aims for sociopolitical change. In the more concrete world of everyday clinical practice, the adoption of a critical perspective means that expert speech-language pathologists seek to critique and evaluate their practice in light of evidence, while at the same time reflecting on the nature of that evidence and its social context and its contribution to the betterment of the services provided to children and adults with communication and swallowing problems.

Critical discourse analysis is one of the approaches to research that has emerged from the critical paradigm. Speech-language pathologists are familiar with discourse analysis as a tool for the assessment of children and adults with language disorders, and many practitioners make use of a discourse framework as the context for intervention. Thus, speech-language pathologists are accustomed to engaging with texts (instances of language produced in natural and meaningful exchanges) through using a range of linguistic analytic methodologies, such as identifying grammatical forms available for the speaker or listener, or identifying macrostructural elements used by the speaker to organize different types of discourse (e.g., narrative or procedural texts). A critical discourse analysis approach integrates such text-based analyses within a framework that incorporates the three critical aspects just outlined—through the analysis of the relationship between texts and sociocultural contexts, through the analysis of how texts reflect and instantiate power relationships, and with the assumption that with greater understanding comes the identification of ways for change to occur. In critical discourse analysis, the detailed text-based analysis is integrated within an analysis of the wider social and cultural discourses in which these texts emerge (and which these texts also serve to produce or maintain). One of the leading linguistic analytic approaches used in critical discourse analysis has been systemic functional linguistics, developed through the work of Halliday and Hasan, and this approach is used in the illustrations of practice—presented in the book. In common with other critical theories, critical discourse analysis also places the examination of power relationships (interpersonal, sociocultural) at the center of explanation and interpretation and explicitly adopts a sociopolitical agenda for change. For example, researchers from a critical discourse

perspective have challenged current orthodoxies with regard to the identification and intervention approaches used for differences in literacy development in light of the influence of socioeconomic factors, and have argued for the importance of explicit teaching of different genres (types of discourse) as a means of empowerment.

This book examines a series of key issues for the expert speech-language pathologist through the lens of critical discourse analysis, in order to offer the opportunity for critical reflection with a view to change. Looking first at practice, the book reconsiders a central and long-standing area for debate among expert practitioners: the validity of assessments. This issue is approached through considering the social context in which speech-language pathology exists and the social roles and functions that speech-language pathologists serve. Subsequently, the book critically examines student learning and curriculum development, taking the view that a primary role for the expert practitioner is that of educator of future speech-language pathologists. A critical perspective is argued to be essential for the educator if we are to avoid "cloning" ourselves and our practices. In every chapter, in order to provide concrete illustration and practical direction for the reader in considering the issues, a number of situations in the area of practice for both children and adults with communication disorders are presented.

Although other works have applied the methodology of discourse analysis to the assessment of clients, and individual contributions appear in chapters in more disorder-focused works that have begun to engage with this paradigm, there has been little recognition of the relevance of the critical approach to professional practice as a whole. This book attempts to address this gap.

The book has been designed to provide advanced-level speech-language pathology theory and practice debate, while introducing the reader to a critical perspective.

Acknowledgments

Writing this book has provided me with an opportunity to bring together the experiences and insights gained through having the opportunity to work with many persons and their families whose lives have been affected by communication disability. This book also has served to crystallize many of the ideas, debates, and discussions in which I have participated over many years with a wide range of scholars, practitioners, and students across diverse fields. To all of these people, too many to name, I owe a considerable debt, which I gratefully acknowledge. Naturally, any misunderstandings or particular biases remain my own. I would like to thank my friends and colleagues in the Clinical Linguistics Research Group for their invaluable contributions to my understanding of how a range of linguistic perspectives, including critical ones, can illuminate our work in speech-language pathology.

To my family
with many thanks for
all their support and encouragement
over the years

1

A Critical Discourse Perspective on Speech-Language Pathology

Discourse as a Reflection of Culture

Expertise typically is seen as a strictly personal attribute of an individual, and much of the research on expert practice has focused on the particular ways in which experts differ from novices with regard to cognition, affect, and psychomotor skills (Higgs & Bithell, 2001). The notion of expertise that emerges throughout this book, however, is that it is socially constructed, created, and reproduced. A critical discourse perspective provides the lens through which expert practice can be viewed as a social construct. Accordingly, no attempt is made here to define expertise at the outset; rather, this different view of expertise unfolds as various aspects and applications of critical discourse analysis are explored throughout the book.

This chapter presents a critical discourse perspective on speech-language pathology, moving beyond those aspects of discourse analysis that are well recognized in the profession to the recognition of the potential contribution of critical discourse analysis as an approach that enables expert practitioners to reflect on their practice. The main conceptual foundations of a critical discourse perspective are outlined first. Examination of expert practice then commences through an analysis of the domain of expertise to which the profession lays claim in documents that set out the scope of practice. It is suggested that notions of appropriateness in communication are fundamental to the identification of the profession's expertise, and yet at the same time, judgments of appropriateness arguably are the most problematic for a critical conception of speech-language pathology practice.

1

Toward a Definition of a Critical Discourse Perspective

Critical discourse is described in the literature variously as a theory, a method, a perspective, and an approach. The term *critical linguistics* usually is applied as an umbrella concept to cover the many diverse linguistic perspectives that embody a critical point of view, whereas *critical discourse* generally covers sociolinguistic perspectives used critically. Use of the term *critical discourse analysis* signals that the methodology for the investigation is based on textual analysis, although such work also may include analysis of broader sociological factors from a range of frameworks. Many introductory reference works are available, designed generally for applied linguists as well as for professionals working in the field of education, and throughout this book, these interdisciplinary insights form a useful counterpoint to the issues that can be identified in speech-language pathology (Locke, 2004; Pennycook, 2001; Rogers, 2004; Young & Harrison, 2004).

This opening section of the chapter outlines the main concepts involved in a critical discourse perspective and examines the relevance of this perspective to speech-language pathology.

"Critical"

The *critical* aspect of a critical discourse perspective encompasses the notion that the explicit goal of the perspective is to reflect on the everyday, taken-for-granted assumptions of social practices involving discourse in order to provide the opportunity for change. One of the dangers of this perspective is that it can be viewed as unnecessarily negative, and certainly the process of such an approach can be very challenging, because it will investigate ideas and practices in which both the researchers and the subjects being studied have considerable personal, professional, and potentially emotional investment. A generally held assumption within critical discourse perspectives, however, is that the spirit of inquiry is essentially positive, aiming to prompt or support some kind of social action for the betterment of those whose lives are affected by whatever it is being studied. This explicit idealistic investment is consistent with the aims of speech-language pathologists, who seek to improve the quality of life for people with communication and swallowing disorders. At the same time, the investment in change clearly biases critical discourse investigations in a particular direction, typically toward problems in which culturally embedded power imbalances can be seen as the central issue.

So, if not "criticism," then, what is meant by *critical*? As an entry point into the diverse approaches within critical theories, it is useful to consider the three main ways of understanding phenomena delineated by Habermas (1972): "The approach of the empirical-analytic sciences incorporates a *technical* cognitive interest; that of the historical-hermeneutic sciences incorporates a *practical* one; and the approach of critically oriented sciences incorporates the *emancipatory* cognitive interest . . . " (p. 308). In line with current terminology, this book uses the following terms to describe these three main ways of understanding the world: *empirical-logical*, as applied in analysis; *interpretive* (integrative), as applied in synthesis; and *reflective* (emancipatory), as applied in critical thinking. *Analysis* provides logical ways of segmenting, categorizing, and deducing information and is associated with modern (or *positivist*) thought. The scientific basis of speech-language pathology is founded on this way of understanding communication phenomena. *Synthesis* provides ways of bringing pieces of information together inductively, to interpret, to theorize as to what the whole might mean, and forms the basis of practical problem-solving. Clinical reasoning in speech-language pathology depends crucially on this way of transforming understanding into action plans. *Critical thinking* provides one further layer, wherein reflection can occur on both analyses and syntheses, from outside the boundaries within which these ways of thinking were framed, with the goal of emancipating people and societies from constraints of knowledge, thinking, and action. Critical approaches have in common a shared view of the relativity of different perspectives on phenomena and generally are seen as *postmodern* or *postpositivist* (although many of the major critical theorists, including Habermas, explicitly reject such labeling).

For example, in a speech-language pathology approach to understanding the sounds of speech, a phonetic and phonemic analysis will provide much information, and from these findings, particular phonological theories are applied and generated to explain how the sounds of speech are made, both in general and in the particular case of a child or adult who is producing sounds differently. In reflecting critically on findings and theories, a speech-language pathologist may ask questions about whether the analysis and theory will hold for the sounds of speech in dialects or other cultures. Furthermore, the speech-language pathologist may question the social and political consequences of applying normative tests of sound production milestones for both an individual child and for the child's cultural peers within the institutional framework of school education. Thus, the "critical" in a critical discourse perspective is all about asking questions, reflecting, and reframing and ideally drives lines of inquiry back through other ways of thinking.

An inherent attention to culture lies within these critical reflections, as both a point of departure (does the phenomenon being studied reflect aspects of culture?) and as a driving force (does the phenomenon being studied create aspects of culture?). Culture within a critical discourse perspective is considered in the broadest sense, in that although it may apply to a particular ethnic culture, it can apply equally to a subculture (for example, teenage gangs or bowling club members). Essentially, culture within a critical discourse perspective refers to groups that share some sense of collective membership within a particular society. Unlike in a line of sociological inquiry, however, it is not general aspects of culture that attract a critical discourse inquiry but particularly those aspects of culture in which issues of power are central to the problems being examined. In one sense, professionals who work within critical discourse perspectives see power as central to all cultural concerns, but this generality arguably is too broad to be helpful for a research focus, so it is the more narrow sense of power relations that focuses critical discourse inquiries. In view of the concerns of the critical discourse perspective with social change, issues of power imbalance and resultant social inequity drive the research focus. These concerns again are consistent with the concerns of speech-language pathology in maximizing social participation for people who experience communication disorders and swallowing disorders, and who face societal barriers and inequities in achieving such participation.

For critical discourse perspectives, one of the major ways in which the operation of power can be seen within cultures is through the examination of the discourses of that culture. One of the axiomatic assumptions within a critical discourse perspective is that specific cultural groups share particular discourses, and that these discourses define, identify, and create the group membership, as discussed next.

"Discourse"

Discourse in a critical discourse perspective is defined broadly in the sense of referring to all of those *types* of talk and writing that are used by members of a culture or society. Although discourse analysts examine particular instances of talk and writing, they are examining them with reference to the type of talk, or the type of writing, of which the instance is an example. Discourse perspectives fall somewhere in between the two extreme views within linguistics, that of language as an abstract conception of the rules for

language reception and formulation (that is, a top-down perspective) and that of "language-in-use," wherein each instance of use is to be examined in its own right (that is, a bottom-up perspective). From the perspective of "language-as-abstract," the proliferation of variation within language-in-use is seen as essentially noise in the system, while from the perspective of language-in-use, the theoretical abstractions do not explain adequately what are seen to be systematic patterns in variation. Perhaps the closest to a true bottom-up perspective is *conversation analysis*, in which instances of language use are seen and analyzed from the participants' perspectives (in the sense of the observable communicative accounts of the participants) for the moment of conversation being examined. Even conversation analysis, however, builds generalizable theories regarding, for example, the general applicability of the turn-taking structures and resources for negotiating understanding and misunderstanding, so it certainly incorporates concerns beyond the instance of language-in-use. Discourse analysis falls somewhere along this continuum, in the sense that it is a sociolinguistic endeavor and therefore remains close to the data of language-in-use and at the same time often is theory-driven.

What constitutes different types of discourse? A diverse array of approaches to this question have been developed, with more or less rigor, within discourse analysis. For example, what one researcher may refer to as a narrative, another may delineate further to describe as a personal recounting, as opposed to a story narrative; or a procedure may be described equally well as just one type of explanation. The terms used to describe types of discourse also are numerous, with *genre* and *text type* among the most common. Each of these terms comes with its own theoretical underpinnings and assumptions. The term *genre* in this book is applied in the sense used in the approach of *systemic functional linguistics*, which allows characterization of the type of discourse in very particular linguistic ways, resulting in a unique configuration of the words and grammar used in association with what is being talked about (for example, the technicality of the vocabulary), with how the language reflects and creates the interpersonal relationship between speaker and listener or writer and reader (for example, the politeness forms used), and with the role of language (for example, whether it is verbal or nonverbal, or whether it constitutes or is ancillary to the interaction) (Halliday & Hasan, 1985). For example, the narrative genre tends to have low-level technical vocabulary, demonstrates considerable use of politeness forms of language to engage the listener or reader, and is verbal or graphic, and wholly constitutes the interaction. By contrast, the exposition genre tends toward higher-level technical vocabulary, uses language to disengage or objectify, may include diagrammatic communication as well as verbal or graphic communication, and may either constitute or partially accompany an interaction.

The term *text type*, on the other hand, generally is associated with theories that relate the generation and understanding of texts to mental models or cognitive schema (Van Dijk, 2006; Van Dijk & Kintsch, 1983), so macrostruc-

tural elements within texts are the important defining features distinguishing different types of texts. For example, although narrative text types may consist of establishing the setting (location, participants, and so on), describing the complicating action, providing a resolution, and optionally a coda, expository text types may consist of establishing the domain, setting out a logical train of points, and providing a conclusion, and optionally a recommendation. In diverse approaches within discourse analysis, however, the terms *genre* and *text type* often are used fairly loosely, and certainly both the lexicogrammatical features and the macrostructural elements are common concerns across many approaches to discourse analysis.

The study of both genre and text types requires data commonly referred to as *texts*, in the practical sense of instances of speaking or writing. A feature of texts is their unity, with their selection guided by observation of moments of talk or writing that "hang together" or form some sort of coherent instance. Any particular text could in fact contain a number of different genres or text types; for example, conversation during a coffee-break may contain examples of narrative discourse (what happened over the weekend), expository discourse (an explanation of a political point of view), and casual chat (such as gossip) (Eggins & Slade, 2004/1997).

Critical discourse inquiries have at their center the study of textual data, and the study of the types of discourse associated with particular cultural contexts. *Context* as used here is another term variously defined by different approaches. Throughout this book, the term is used to allow movement from the general construct of culture to the particular instantiation of culture in a particular situation. So, for example, in considering the culture of hospitals, a particular inquiry may focus more narrowly on particular contexts (for practical purposes, even if for no other reason)—the inquiry may look more closely at case conferences in order to examine professional interactions within the hospital culture. The *context of situation* is another construct very much associated with systemic functional linguistics, which is very specifically described with reference to the *field* of discourse (what is being talked about), the *tenor* of discourse (the role relationship between interactants), and the *mode* of discourse (the role of language within that context) (Halliday & Hasan, 1985). This dialectic, between the cultural context and the discourses associated with it, is another key assumption within a critical discourse perspective. The term *dialectic* implies a two-way interaction between cultural contexts and types of discourse such that the cultural context shapes (dictates or constrains) the types of discourse considered to be allowable or appropriate within that context, while at the same time, the types of discourse shape or change the cultural context (the notion of appropriateness is revisited later in the chapter). For example, an argument with a client is an unexpected type of discourse within a typical therapy session, so such nonstandard discourse in this context will have consequences for the interaction, generating a shift in the role relationship between therapist and client and challenging cultural assumptions (Simmons-Mackie & Damico, 1999).

"Analysis"

If a critical discourse perspective involves studying and reflecting on the types of discourse used within cultural contexts, then the final aspect to be considered is that of *analysis*. Diverse methodologies are used to conduct such analyses, with some inquiries using broad sociological and sociolinguistic constructs, others using ethnography and ethnomethodologically inspired qualitative analyses (including conversation analysis), and still others making use of linguistic methods of discourse analysis (Kress, 1990). Although a range of linguistic analyses have been applied, one of the most useful and widely applied within critical discourse perspectives is that of systemic functional linguistics (Halliday & Matthiessen, 2004). This linguistic model is a top-down approach to language-in-use that seeks to describe and explain the dialectical relationship between context and text—that is, between culture as encapsulated within contexts of situation and the levels of language used in texts (phonological and gestural expression, lexicogrammar, discourse-semantic levels of language). The application of systemic functional linguistics to empirical studies of discourse has provided critical discourse inquiries with systematic and replicable methodological tools. Of the examples presented in this book, many make use of systemic functional linguistics, although both broader qualitative analyses as well as conversation analysis also are used. Chapter 9 returns to these diverse methodologies and considers their relative contributions for a critical discourse perspective on speech-language pathology.

To summarize, a critical discourse perspective is concerned with shedding light on power relations in cultures, as revealed and instantiated through discourse, and in promoting change to alleviate social inequities associated with power imbalances. This perspective is critical in the sense of considering and reflecting on ideas and practice embedded within cultural contexts and uses the study of types of discourse as the relevant artifacts for this consideration, making use of a range of methodologies including sociolinguistic approaches to analyze the discourse.

A Critical Discourse Perspective on Scope of Practice

The most fundamental question that can be asked regarding speech-language pathology is "What is the domain of expertise within the field?" It is possible, for example, to consider the expertise of speech-language pathologists from the point of view of the "person-in-the-street" (and such research is discussed in Chapter 9). For the moment, however, by way of an entry point to thinking within a critical discourse perspective, this discussion focuses on the profession's ideas regarding its domain of expertise. Statements about scope of practice in speech-language pathology are a source of textual data that encapsulate the profession's view of itself. Such statements usually contain some explicit declaration of their purpose, generally aiming to provide information to the general public, potential employers, and clients and their care-

givers regarding what they can expect a speech-language pathologist to do. These statements are put together through the work of members and employees of the associations that represent the profession and are available to the general public in a number of countries. In view of the time and effort that go into producing these documents, it is possible to be confident that the wording has been given close attention by the writers and that these writers are experts in the field; hence, these artifacts are of particular interest from a critical discourse perspective as a way of unpacking the sociocultural meanings conveyed in these texts. The following discussion is based on the examination of statements of scope of practice available on the websites for the American Speech-Language-Hearing Association (ASHA) (www.asha.org), the Canadian Association of Speech-Language Pathologists and Audiologists (CASLPA) (www.caslpa.ca), and the Speech Pathology Association of Australia (SPAA) (www.speechpathology australia.org.au). Each of these associations provides a particular document identified as the profession's statement with regard to scope of practice.

The first point of interest from a critical discourse perspective is in the description of the nature of the problems with which speech-language pathologists are concerned. Both ASHA and SPAA statements explicitly draw on the World Health Organization (WHO) framework (WHO, 2001) in order to describe communication and swallowing with reference to impairment of bodily functions, limitations on communication and swallowing activity, and restrictions of social participation in relation to communication and swallowing. The ASHA statement provides the more detailed description of scope of practice in this regard:

> The scope of practice in speech-language pathology encompasses all components and factors identified in the WHO framework. That is, speech-language pathologists work to improve quality of life by reducing impairments of body functions and structures, activity limitations, participation restrictions, and environmental barriers of the individuals they serve. They serve individuals with known disease processes (e.g., aphasia, cleft palate) as well as those with activity limitations or participation restrictions (e.g., individuals needing classroom support services or special educational placement), including when such limitations or restrictions occur in the absence of known disease processes or impairments (e.g. individuals with differences in dialect). The role of speech-language pathologists includes prevention of communication, swallowing, or other upper aerodigestive disorders as well as diagnosis, habilitation, rehabilitation, and enhancement of these functions. (ASHA, 2001, p. 1–28)

The WHO framework used here attempts to circumvent terminology and taxonomic classifications that have become stigmatized over the years— for example, the replacement of the concept of handicap, which was an important step forward in the 1980s in the recognition of social restrictions that could occur independently of impairment, with the concept of restrictions on social participation. Accordingly, the current terminology could be seen as "politically correct" terminology. Of

interest, in more recent years, the term *politically correct* has come to be used pejoratively, with some backlash against the use of terms seen to be used euphemistically. Such debates regarding the social acceptability of terms, however, represent just the surface of a critical discourse inquiry. Of greater interest here is the clear identification that speech-language pathologists are concerned with difficulties that arise as a result of speech and language difference or variation. This point opens the issues surrounding how judgments can be made and when the determination of difference and variation is appropriate or not. This issue of appropriateness is central to practice in speech-language pathology and is taken up later in this chapter.

The statements of scope of practice identify the speech-language pathologist as the active agent, with relative "backgrounding" of the person with a communication or swallowing disorder or difficulty. In these documents, speech-language pathologists *do* things —for example, "assess," "treat," and so on—whereas people with communication and swallowing disorders are passive recipients of actions instigated by speech-language pathologists. Person-first description of people with communication disorder is increasingly in use in line with current debates and concerns with regard to how to describe the populations involved. This person-first terminology provides greater potential for agentive forms than if just disorder types were listed. For example, such terminology means that it would be possible to state: "Individuals with communication disorders can contact speech-language pathologists directly for services"—but in fact no instances exist in any of these documents in which persons with communication or swallowing disorders or difficulties are agentive. The relative invisibility of such persons in relation to the professional in these documents becomes more apparent when it is noted that speech-language pathologists either "provide services for" or "serve" people in these populations. A striking finding is that in these documents, "collaboration" occurs only between speech-language pathologists and other professionals who similarly "provide services." The closest characterization of working partnerships with persons with communication and swallowing disorders or difficulties comes with the identification of "family-centered approaches" and the description of "working with" people in these populations in the SPAA document (SPAA, 2002). From a critical discourse perspective, these observations point to a fundamental imbalance in the power relationship between professionals and people with communication and swallowing disorders.

A more detailed examination of the wording in these documents is possible through a taxonomic analysis (Martin & Rose, 2003, p. 103), which reveals that, as might be expected, a large proportion (32%) of terms used in these documents are highly specialized and technical. For example, concrete specialized terms such as "cleft palate" or "augmentative and alternative communication devices," as well as abstract technical terms such as "phonology," "morphology," "semantics," and "syntax," are used. Additionally, the relationship between speech-language

pathology and the social institutions in which it is embedded is revealed through the incorporation of abstract institutional terms such as "service delivery models," "local, state, and national levels," and "outcomes measurement activities."

Another feature of interest in these scope of practice documents is the tension between a very plain-English use of active verbs to describe what speech-language pathologists do ("identify, define, and diagnose," "educate, supervise, and mentor," and so on, which is most notable in the ASHA document) and the adoption of a writing style commonly associated with scientific writing, involving heavy use of *nominalization* (Halliday, 1985/1989). Nominalization is described within systemic functional linguistics as an ideational metaphor wherein one type of language is used for another; in this case, a process becomes a thing (Martin & Rose, 2003, pp. 103–107). Nominalization essentially renders active verbs into static nouns—for example, *prevent* becomes *prevention*, and so on. These metaphorical entities make up 50% of all of the different kinds of entities referred to in the scope of practice documents. All three documents use the following terms to describe the processes involved in speech-language pathology: *identify, treat, educate, counsel, prevent, manage, assess, refer,* and *rehabilitate*. In all three documents, these terms are nominalized. Two other terms are used to describe processes in the three documents: *enhance* and *research*; these are nominalized in two of the three documents. None of the documents use the terms 'counsel', 'prevent', and 'rehabilitate' as verbs;

that is, these terms always appear in nominalized form (*counseling, prevention, rehabilitation*).

Nominalization is a stylistic device that can be seen as serving social purposes—for example, to raise the status of the writing. This aspect of scientific writing style not only is seen in published documents but infiltrates spoken scientific presentations, again with associations of higher status within the social community of such events (Rowley-Jolivet & Carter-Thomas, 2005). On looking at the scope of practice documents from a critical discourse perspective, then, it can be asked what are the social messages sent (and received by target audiences) by the use of such stylistic devices. A possible result of use of such devices (and only one possibility) is the shift of focus from what is done as a process to the provision of a product—for example, speech-language pathologists provide a product called "screening," and so on. Such language choices are rarely conscious, but the product focus may be seen as reflecting important current social movements of corporatization of health and education services, involving, among other things, a consumer or customer focus (rather than a focus on patients, clients, or people) and a delineation of particular markets for these services. In other words, through this product focus, the profession identifies what others can purchase or use. Within this wider social movement of corporatization (Fairclough, 2004), such a linguistic convention may be considered to be strategic for the profession. Possibly, however, the strategy also may be seen to contribute to the relative invisibility of the person with a communication or swallowing difficulty or disorder.

Of course, the social purpose in relation to the aspect of scope in these documents is not just to state what it is that speech-language pathologists do, or with whom they work, but to delineate the boundaries of practice. The statement of the territory within the boundaries is very broad, with no explicit statements as to what is done by speech-language pathologists rather than by others. Through such wide-ranging claims for territory, these documents attempt to provide a resource for speech-language pathologists to use in particular instances. As insiders, members of the profession can recognize perhaps where these territorial justifications are implicit in the documents, such as in statements regarding speech-language pathologists' role in case management and financial administration, and in statements regarding use of instrumentation, such as video-endoscopy, in which requirements for specialized training are noted. On the other hand, the statement of what lies outside the boundaries is more explicit, particularly with regard to hearing, probably because of the historically close association between audiology and speech-language pathology training and practice—for example, "This does not include sensory devices used by individuals with hearing loss or other auditory perceptual devices" (ASHA, 2001, section 6, p. 1–29). Other statements regarding what lies outside the boundaries are more implicit and possibly require an insider to notice the fine distinctions being made—for example, "Counselling on aspects of communication, swallowing disorders and therapy" (SPAA, 2002, p. 2) and "Screening of hearing and other factors for the purpose of speech-language evaluation" (CASLPA, 1998, p. 1). An alternative way to identify the boundaries that speech-language pathologists are not to cross is through statements of when referral to other professionals is required, although these professionals are relatively underspecified—for example, " . . . evaluation of esophageal function is for the purpose of referral to medical professionals" (ASHA, 2001, section 1, p. 1–28).

All three documents stress that scope of practice can be expected to change over the course of time and thereby implicitly acknowledge the role of historical sociocultural context in shaping practice, while at the same time providing a gap in the fence, as it were, for territorial expansion. The way in which boundaries shift raises important questions that warrant further attention in the field. The scope of practice documents themselves provide textual artifacts that signal the points at which these boundary shifts may be occurring. As Wenger and colleagues have discussed in relation to communities of practice, well-accepted practices require no special justification or debate, because these practices constitute assumed knowledge within and outside the particular community, but boundary disputes and justifications are required when practices are changing (Wenger, 1998; Wenger, McDermott, & Snyder, 2002). In the scope of practice documents, it can be seen that expert practice drives change, as, for example, when specialized training in particular techniques becomes, first, a possibility for some practitioners and then, over time, a fundamental requirement of professional preparation (a sociohistorical account of the rise of dysphagia practice would provide such

an illustrative case example). On the other hand, what might be seen as non-expert practice also drives change. For example, the Royal College of Speech and Language Therapists (www.rcslt.org) embeds much of its statements with regard to scope of practice within a range of pivotal documents, but the most explicit delineation of scope of practice is found within its documents outlining the work of support personnel, in order to attempt to clearly delineate the limitations of the role of such personnel in relation to that of a qualified speech-language pathologist (*RCSLT competencies project support practitioner framework*, 2002).

In summary, then, thus far it has been suggested that speech-language pathology practice reflects its sociocultural and sociohistorical context, and a critical analysis of the discourses produced by the profession in relation to scope of practice has shed some light on past, present, and future practices. As previously mentioned, however, scope of practice involves tackling the notion of appropriateness of communication, and this notion has a major role in identifying the specific expertise of the profession.

A Critical Perspective on the Notion of Appropriateness

The term *appropriateness of communication* came into prominence in the field of speech-language pathology during the 1980s, associated with a significant theoretical paradigm shift influenced by linguistic perspectives on pragmatics. Pragmatics in linguistics refers to a perspective which seeks to understand language-in-use, and which developed with substantial influence from philosophical thought regarding how meaning could come to be created. As Prutting (1982) has discussed, in speech-language pathology, pragmatics was seen less as a perspective on language use (Levinson, 1983) and more as a layer of analysis, such that as well as analyzing communication in terms of layers of phonology, morphology and syntax, and semantics, speech-language pathologists also looked at social communication under the rubric of pragmatics. The development was important in providing a theoretically informed approach to what had hitherto been a common-sense, yet rather ad hoc approach to understanding "functional" communication. Speech-language pathologists applied the work on speech act theory of Austin (1975) and Searle (1969) to describe and classify the different functional purposes to which children and adults with communication disorders used language. Grice's (1975) discussion of implicature (i.e. how inferential meaning is exchanged) and its relationship with assumed maxims of quantity, quality, relevance, and efficiency were applied by Damico in a framework to analyze classroom interaction (Damico, 1985), although later developments in relevance theory (Sperber & Wilson, 1986, 1995; Wilson & Sperber, 2004) were not taken up in the field. Both Prutting and Kirchner (1983, 1987) and Penn (1985, 1987) drew from a range of pragmatic approaches to develop clinically useful checklists and rating scales to describe the language use of children and adults with language disorders. Their work brought to prominence the

use of appropriateness as an alternative description to correctness when describing the differences observed in language use. For speech-language pathologists, the term *appropriateness* allowed for explicit recognition of the importance of looking at communicative adequacy in situations in which accuracy was not achieved. Appropriateness could then be recognized as a legitimate goal of therapy and prompted the development of therapies such as PACE (Promoting Aphasics' Communicative Effectiveness) (Davis & Wilcox, 1981; Glindemann & Springer, 1995). In what Duchan and colleagues describe as the second stage of the development of applications of pragmatics in speech-language pathology, the importance of integrating natural contexts into both assessment and interventions came to be increasingly recognized (Duchan, Hewitt, & Sonnenmeier, 1994).

This foundational work underpins much current research. In the area of acquired adult neurogenic disorders, Prutting and Kirchner's pragmatic protocol has been applied to describe the appropriateness of communication in persons with Parkinson's disease, successfully identifying those with frontal lobe involvement (McNamara & Durso, 2003), and a modified form has been applied to describe the appropriateness of communication in persons with left and right cerebrovascular accidents in describing emotional experiences (Borod et al., 2000), and Penn's protocol has been applied to the study of primary progressive aphasia and frontal lobe dementia (Orange, Kertesz, & Peacock, 1998). In the area of child language disorders, pragmatics continues to inform child language assessment and intervention (Camarata, 2000). Indeed, pragmatics itself has come to describe a type of communication impairment, because the social communication difficulties commonly observed in children with high-functioning autism spectrum disorders were described initially as exhibiting semantic-pragmatic disorder, and more recently as having pragmatic language impairment (Bishop & Norbury, 2002). Common to both past and current work within pragmatic perspectives is an assumption that speech-language pathologists are able to make valid judgments regarding appropriateness of communication. Tests of validity of these judgments have been constrained to reports of intra- and interjudge reliability, so that if two speech-language pathologists agree with each other and themselves, then this has been considered sufficient evidence of validity. Difficulties obtaining adequate levels of interjudge agreement are reported as methodological limitations (Coelho, Youse, & Le, 2002), rather than considered as raising more fundamental questions regarding the validity of the descriptive measures themselves. A few studies have compared ratings of appropriateness of speech-language pathologists with those of others, but differences between expert and lay judgment have been interpreted as indicating faulty judgment of the nonexpert or as potentially confounded by the cognitive limitations associated with the disorder (Channon & Watts, 2003). The assumed expertise of speech-language pathologists in making judgments of appropriateness is such that they have been used as experts in judging the communication of other professionals' interaction with people with communication disorders (McConkey, Morris, & Purcell, 1999).

The validity of speech-language pathologists' judgments of appropriateness, however, can be questioned on a number of grounds. The profession itself is built on the societal recognition that for some people, communication is sufficiently inaccurate or different to be, first, labeled as disordered and, second, identified as requiring someone to do something about this difference. The profession thus has an implicit investment in the association of difference with disorder. The theories that inform an understanding of communication disorders are deficit-oriented, in that analysis relies on detection of difference. Speech-language pathologists working within sociolinguistic and pragmatic perspectives argue for the need to separate analytic steps of detection and description of difference from interpretive steps of attribution of disorder (Prutting & Kirchner, 1983), but even with methodological safeguards it is difficult to avoid the conflation of observed difference with the construct of deficit. Even in the area of stuttering, in which identification and measurement could be argued to have been more developed than in the study of language disorders, similar debates emerge. For example, debate continues regarding the frequency and nature of disfluency that may prompt the average listener or the affected person to describe the phenomenon as stuttering (Ingham & Cordes, 1997; Lickley, Hartsuiker, Corley, Russell, & Nelson, 2005). Even when the disorder is clearly present (through documented medical case history for example), is every instance of difference reflective of the disorder, or do some instances represent just an everyday slip of the tongue? This debate can become unproductively circular, but this does not remove the question or the importance of its implications for an understanding of the nature of communication disorders. The validity of speech-language pathologists' judgments regarding appropriateness also is questionable in light of their extensive experience with communication disorders, because this provides them with background knowledge that is not shared by other members of the community. Although expert speech-language pathologists may confidently rate a person's disorder as mild, moderate, or severe in a way that reflects the distribution of severity across the range of a particular disorder, these gradings may not reflect either the experience and perceptions of the affected person or those of the people with whom that person interacts. Recent research into the prevalence of stuttering, voice and speech-sound disorders in children (McKinnon, McLeod, & Reilly, 2007) suggests that the reasons why teachers' identification of disorders may be considered both valid and reliable include their ability to make multiple observations across a range of performance tasks and to compare the performance with that of a normally distributed population. Although the investigators note that teachers' rate for identification of disorders typically is lower than that of speech-language pathologists, they remain silent on possible reasons for this discrepancy. At the very least, the theoretical debate and the practical concerns raised regarding the deficit basis of speech-language pathology prompt the question "Who else thinks so?" with respect to appropriateness and suggest that comprehensive analysis

should be accompanied by cautious interpretation.

Locked into the notion of appropriateness is the question "Appropriate for what?" This question signals the importance of the recognition of context within pragmatic approaches. In other words, although accuracy can be seen as possible to judge with reference to some normative or prescribed standard, appropriateness necessarily is judged in relation to the contextual demands of the social and communicative situation. Accuracy and notions of error, however, are just as context-bound as notions of appropriateness. The context in which accuracy and error are judged is the known limits or range of typical performance, or the societal construct of the "right" or standard way in which language is used. Appropriateness seems a more "fuzzy" concept, perhaps because a greater range of typical performance is observed in the types of language to which it is applied—for example, humor or sarcasm. The context-bound nature of both error and appropriateness becomes evident when it is considered how much both are influenced by the most obvious sociological influences, that of gender and education. Rather than fighting against these constructs, it is suggested that through embracing the relevant aspects of contextual variation and influence, speech-language pathologists can work toward an adequate description of communication disorder.

Figure 1–1 describes the key dimensions of context widely recognized as pivotal for the exchange of meaning (Halliday & Hasan, 1985; Halliday & Matthiessen, 2004; Lickley et al., 2005), and for an understanding of appropri-

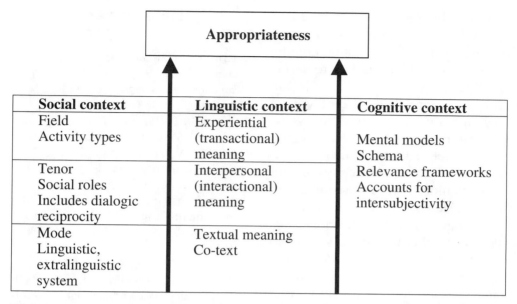

| Appropriateness | | |

Social context	Linguistic context	Cognitive context
Field Activity types	Experiential (transactional) meaning	Mental models Schema Relevance frameworks Accounts for intersubjectivity
Tenor Social roles Includes dialogic reciprocity	Interpersonal (interactional) meaning	
Mode Linguistic, extralinguistic system	Textual meaning Co-text	

Figure 1–1. Appropriateness and context. (Based on Fetzer & Ackman, 2002; Halliday & Matthiessen, 2004; Van Dijk, 2006.)

ateness of communication in context (Fetzer & Akman, 2002). The thick dark lines on the diagram are used to illustrate that these interfaces between social and linguistic context, and between linguistic and cognitive context, are threads that interweave to make up the complex fabric of appropriateness. It is possible to unravel this fabric in order to see the patterns that emerge along these interfaces. For example, different social roles in the context of situation are associated with certain linguistic interpersonal roles, as when the social role of lecturer allows for extended monologic discourse to be seen as entirely appropriate (which it would not be for the same person in the social role of spouse). Particular cognitive schemata, such as having a meal in a restaurant, are associated with specific types of discourse, and relevance theory may explain why, for

example, talking about being short of money may raise questions in the listener-diner regarding who will be paying for the meal! Appropriateness in communication is not a feature of one or the other participant but rather emerges from the shared understanding of all participants involved; accordingly, much that could be said may be left unsaid and specific meanings can still be conveyed.

A critical discourse perspective raises questions regarding the inherent dangers in how the notion of appropriateness is applied. Fairclough challenges approaches to teaching language which use notions of appropriateness in language use as skills or competencies to be trained and developed (Fairclough, 1995). He argues that models of appropriateness are based on faulty models of language variation, in that they assume a closely defined relationship between different types of language use and particular contexts, that these are in general use in most situations by most speakers, that it is easy to decide whether language use is or is not appropriate, and that different types of language use are easy to differentiate. Fairclough argues that these assumptions are not sustainable, in view of the range of variation within any community, situation, type of discourse, and speaker. He also argues that the use of appropriateness as an educational goal is really an attitude or, more strongly, a declaration of the political ideology of the users, such that the aim is for maintenance of a conservative social order as reflected in and created by language use. Instead, Fairclough argues for the importance of promoting a critical awareness in language learners of the social choices involved in different uses of language, and that understanding appropriateness provides a way to involve learners in actively making creative use of language for their ends. The relevance of this critical perspective to speech-language pathology relates to the previously discussed issue of the validity of speech-language pathologists' judgements as to appropriateness because this becomes a pivotal theoretical stance, with some very concrete methodological implications. Working with people with communication disorders to facilitate their knowledge and skills in order to unpack the key elements of appropriateness in language use becomes a key goal, and the assessment process changes from the judgment of another person's language use to a dynamic co-discovery of how that person is using language for what ends and with what outcomes.

References

American Speech-Language-Hearing Association. (2001). *Scope of practice in speech-language pathology*. Rockville, MD: Author.

Austin, J. L. (1975). *How to do things with words*. Oxford: Clarendon Press.

Bishop, D. V., & Norbury, C. N. (2002). Exploring the borderlands of autistic disorder and specific language impairment: A study using standardised diagnostic instruments. *Journal of Child Psychology & Psychiatry & Allied Disciplines, 43*(7), 917–929.

Borod, J. C., Rorie, K. D., Pick, L. H., Bloom, R. L., Andelman, F., Campbell, A. L., et al. (2000). Verbal pragmatics following unilateral stroke: Emotional content and valence. *Neuropsychology, 14*(1), 112–124.

Camarata, S. M. (2000). The pragmatics of paediatric language intervention: Issues and analysis. In N. Muller (Ed.), *Pragmatics and speech and language pathology* (pp. 139–163). Amsterdam: John Benjamins.

Canadian Association of Speech-Language Pathologists and Audiologists. (1998). *Scopes of practice in speech-language pathology and audiology in Canada*. Ottawa: Author.

Channon, S., & Watts, M. (2003). Pragmatic language interpretation after closed head injury: Relationship to executive functioning. *Cognitive Neuropsychiatry, 8*(4), 243–260.

Coelho, C., Youse, K. M., & Le, K. N. (2002). Conversational discourse in closed-head-injured and non-brain-injured adults. *Aphasiology, 16*(4/5/6), 659–672.

Damico, J. S. (1985). Clinical discourse analysis: A functional approach to language assessment. In C. S. Simon (Ed.), *Communication skills and classroom success: Assessment of language learning disabled students*. San Diego, CA: College-Hill.

Davis, G. A., & Wilcox, M. J. (1981). Incorporating parameters of natural conversation in aphasia treatment. In R. Chapey (Ed.), *Language intervention strategies in adult aphasia*. Baltimore: Williams & Wilkins.

Duchan, J. F., Hewitt, L. E., & Sonnenmeier, R. M. (1994). Three themes: Stage two pragmatics, combating marginalization, and the relation of theory and practice. In J. F. Duchan, L. E. Hewitt, & R. M. Sonnenmeier (Eds.), *Pragmatics: From theory to practice* (pp. 1–9). Englewood Cliffs, NJ: Prentice-Hall.

Eggins, S., & Slade, D. (2004/1997). *Analysing casual conversation*. London/New York: Equinox/Cassell.

Fairclough, N. (1995). The appropriacy of 'appropriateness'. In *Critical discourse analysis: The critical study of language* (pp. 233–252). London: Longman.

Fairclough, N. (2004). Critical discourse analysis in researching language in the new capitalism: Overdetermination, transdisciplinarity, and textual analysis. In L. Young & C. Harrison (Eds.), *Systemic functional linguistics and critical discourse analysis* (pp. 103–122). London: Continuum.

Fetzer, A., & Akman, V. (2002). Contexts of social action: Guest editors' introduction. *Language & Communication, 22,* 391–402.

Glindemann, R., & Springer, L. (1995). The assessment of PACE therapy. In C. Code & D. Muller (Eds.), *The treatment of aphasia: From theory to practice* (pp. 90–107). London: Whurr.

Grice, H. P. (1975). Logic and conversation. In P. Cole & J. L. Morgan (Eds.), *Syntax and semantics: Vol. 3, Speech acts* (pp. 41–58). New York: Academic Press.

Habermas, J. (1972). *Knowledge and human interests* (J. J. Shapiro, Trans.). London: Heinemann Educational.

Halliday, M. A. K. (1985). *Spoken and written language*. Geelong, Victoria, Australia: Deakin University Press

Halliday, M. A. K., & Hasan, R. (Eds.). (1985). *Language, context, and text: Aspects of language in a social-semiotic perspective*. Geelong, Victoria, Australia: Deakin University.

Halliday, M. A. K., & Matthiessen, C. M. I. M. (2004). *An introduction to functional grammar* (3rd ed.). London: Arnold.

Higgs, J., & Bithell, C. (2001). Professional expertise. In J. Higgs & A. Titchen (Eds.), *Practice knowledge and expertise in the health professions* (pp. 59–68). Oxford: Butterworth Heinemann.

Ingham, R. J., & Cordes, A. K. (1997). Identifying the authoritative judgments of stuttering: Comparisons of self-judgments and observer judgments. *Journal of Speech, Language, and Hearing Research, 40*(3), 581–594.

Kress, G. (1990). Critical discourse analysis. *Annual Review of Applied Linguistics, 11,* 84–99.

Levinson, S. C. (1983). *Pragmatics*. London: Cambridge University Press.

Lickley, R. J., Hartsuiker, R. J., Corley, M., Russell, M., & Nelson, R. (2005). Judgment of disfluency in people who stutter and people who do not stutter: Results from magnitude estimation. *Language and Speech, 48*(3), 299–312.

Locke, T. (2004). *Critical discourse analysis*. London: Continuum.

Martin, J. R., & Rose, D. (2003). *Working with discourse: Meaning beyond the clause*. London: Continuum.

McConkey, R., Morris, I., & Purcell, M. (1999). Communications between staff and adults with intellectual disabilities in naturally occurring settings. *Journal of Intellectual Disability Research, 43*(3), 194–205.

McKinnon, D. H., McLeod, S., & Reilly, S. (2007). The prevalence of stuttering, voice, and speech-sound disorders in primary school students in Australia. *Language, Speech, and Hearing Services in Schools, 38,* 5–15.

McNamara, P., & Durso, R. (2003). Pragmatic communication skills in patients with Parkinson's disease. *Brain and Language, 84,* 414–423.

Orange, J. B., Kertesz, A., & Peacock, J. (1998). Pragmatics in frontal lobe dementia and primary progressive aphasia. *Journal of Neurolinguistics, 11*(1–2), 153–177.

Penn, C. (1985). The profile of communicative appropriateness: A clinical tool for the assessment of pragmatics. *South African Journal of Communication Disorders, 32,* 18–23.

Penn, C. (1987). Compensation and language recovery in the chronic aphasic patient. *Aphasiology, 1*(3), 235–245.

Pennycook, A. (2001). *Critical applied linguistics: A critical introduction.* Mahwah, NJ: Lawrence Erlbaum.

Prutting, C. A. (1982). Pragmatics as social competence. *Journal of Speech & Hearing Disorders, 47,* 123–134.

Prutting, C. A., & Kirchner, D. M. (1983). Applied pragmatics. In T. M. Gallagher & C. A. Prutting (Eds.), *Pragmatic assessment and intervention issues in language.* San Diego, CA: College-Hill.

Prutting, C. A., & Kirchner, D. M. (1987). A clinical appraisal of the pragmatic aspects of language. *Journal of Speech and Hearing Disorders, 52*(2), 105–119.

RCSLT competencies project support practitioner framework. (2002). Retrieved January 7, 2007, from http://www.rcslt.org/docs/competencies_framework.pdf

Rogers, R. (Ed.). (2004). *An introduction to critical discourse analysis in education.* Mahwah, NJ: Lawrence Erlbaum.

Rowley-Jolivet, E., & Carter-Thomas, S. (2005). Genre awareness and rhetorical appropriacy: Manipulation of information structure by NS and NNS scientists in the international conference setting. *English for Specific Purposes, 24,* 41–64.

Searle, J. R. (1969). *Speech acts.* London: Cambridge University Press.

Simmons-Mackie, N., & Damico, J. S. (1999). Social role negotiation in aphasia therapy: Competence, incompetence, and conflict. In D. Kovarsky, J. F. Duchan & M. Maxwell (Eds.), *Constructing (in)competence: Disabling evaluations in clinical and social interaction* (pp. 313–342). Mahwah, NJ: Lawrence Erlbaum.

Speech Pathology Association of Australia. (2002). *Scope of practice in speech pathology.* Melbourne, Victoria, Australia: Author.

Sperber, D., & Wilson, D. (1986). *Relevance: Communication and cognition.* Oxford: Blackwell.

Sperber, D., & Wilson, D. (1995). *Relevance: Communication and cognition* (2nd ed.). Oxford: Blackwell.

Van Dijk, T. A. (2006). Discourse, context and cognition. *Discourse Studies, 8*(1), 159–177.

Van Dijk, T. A., & Kintsch, W. (1983). *Strategies of discourse comprehension.* New York: Academic Press.

Wenger, E. (1998). *Communities of practice: Learning, meaning, and identity.* Cambridge: Cambridge University Press.

Wenger, E., McDermott, R., & Snyder, W. M. (2002). *Cultivating communities of practice: A guide to managing knowledge.* Boston: Harvard Business School Press.

Wilson, D., & Sperber, D. (2004). Relevance theory. In L. R. Horn & G. Ward (Eds.), *The handbook of pragmatics* (pp. 607–632). Malden, MA: Blackwell

World Health Organization. (2001). *ICF: International classification of functioning, disability and health.* Geneva: Author.

Young, L., & Harrison, C. (Eds.). (2004). *Systemic functional linguistics and critical discourse analysis.* London: Continuum.

2

The Focus of Assessment: Layers of Discourse, Layers of Thinking

This chapter reviews assessment practices in speech-language pathology in the light of a critical perspective. First, the recurring debates within the discipline regarding issues that affect the validity of assessment are reviewed, and the sociopolitical context of these debates is considered. Concerns about validity often are countered by suggestions to use multiple sources of data, so a second focus of this chapter is on the notion of triangulation. It is argued that the interpretive stance offered through triangulation is a prominent feature of expert clinical decision-making and at the same time a highly contextualized process. Third, different assessment practices for determining and reporting outcomes and efficacy in the current paradigm of evidence-based practice are reviewed (see also Chapter 8). It is further argued that expert practitioners have a social responsibility for how assessment practices are shaped by sociopolitical pressures, and directions for further research and considerations in this area are discussed.

Throughout the chapter, the multilayered nature of discourse is emphasized, along with the need to attend to each level in order to gain a full perspective. Each act of communication, whether it directly involves or is about someone with communication difficulty, is seen as multilayered in simultaneously being about something (i.e., field), occurring between interactants (i.e., tenor), and using language (i.e., mode) for its enactment (Halliday & Matthiessen, 2004). Each act of communication also can be seen as taking place within an immediately personal context, a local community context, and a broader sociocultural context, and looking at each of these three levels of context offers additional layers of insight into the communication. Also, in attempting to understand communication, the three main ways of thinking drawn from the work of Habermas (introduced in Chapter 1)—analysis, synthesis, and critique—offer three corresponding layers of understanding (Habermas, 1972).

Validity of Assessment

Validity of assessment is of both theoretical and practical significance to speech-language pathologists, in attempting to understand the nature of communication difficulty in general terms, as well as to understand the particular communication difficulties faced by the affected person. Much of the work in this area that informs the practice of speech-language pathology comes from the discipline of psychology in its development of the notions of face validity, construct validity, concurrent validity, and so on (Kazdin, 2003).

Discussed next are two main issues that have proved to be of ongoing concern and debate within speech-language pathology: (1) the contexts of sampling (and inherently within this concern, the methods or process of sampling) and (2) the aspects of discourse selected for analysis and interpretation.

Contexts of Sampling

In the professional discourse about assessment in speech-language pathology, probably one of the most frequently discussed dichotomies is that between the need for controlled conditions of sampling and the need for sampling under natural conditions.

Controlled conditions of sampling are held to be needed in order to identify factors that affect communication, and to test systematically the influence of such selected factors. Controlling the conditions of sampling aims to allow for repeated testing so that any changes associated with development, recovery, or response to therapy can be ascer-

tained. The limitation of controlled conditions of sampling, however, is the difficulty of preserving all of the features of natural, everyday communication contexts. When assessment is conducted under non-natural conditions, then researchers and clinicians need to consider ecological *validity*, that is, the extent to which they can compare test performance with real-world performance (Banerjee & Luoma, 1997; Chaytor & Schmitter-Edgecombe, 2003).

Natural conditions of sampling are held to be needed so that clinician-researchers can observe instances of communication that are authentic and fully represent the nature of difficulties experienced by the affected person (Marquardt & Gillam, 1999). Degrees of naturalness also are considered to influence validity. For example, Vanhalle and colleagues (2000) compared 14 persons with right hemisphere brain damage and 14 matched control subjects on three tasks: natural (a simulated medical-style interview with set questions involving a balanced set of direct and indirect speech acts), non-natural (a task in which the person had to select the most appropriate of four responses to direct and indirect speech acts prompted by a scenario), and pseudonatural (which set up the same sort of tasks as for the non-natural one, but using a medical-style interview as the prompting scenario). These investigators found that both groups of participants did significantly better in responding to indirect speech acts on the natural tasks. Persons with right hemisphere brain damage did no worse than control subjects, on average, in both the natural and the pseudonatural tasks; persons with right hemisphere brain damage showed more difficulty only in the non-natural task. The investigators concluded that their findings raise considerable questions regarding the extent to which previously reported difficulties with indirect speech acts of persons with right hemisphere brain damage may constitute an artifact of non-natural task elicitation demands (Vanhalle et al., 2000).

Degrees of naturalness also are present within data collection in natural settings. Bornstein and colleagues recorded the utterances of 30 two-year-olds in three different natural sampling conditions—sole play (at home, mother in room, with researchers video recording), play with mother (at home, with researchers video recording), and an optimal audio recording carried out by the mother at a time she decided the child produced most and best language (Bornstein, Painter, & Park, 2002). Although correlations in performance were found in all of the conditions, the optimal condition produced the most utterances and the most complex language. The findings of this research underscore the effects of observers in obtaining data, even under everyday eliciting conditions, and the value of parent-assisted data collection in obtaining natural samples raises important questions regarding alternative methods of time-effective and valid natural data collection (Bornstein et al.).

Facets of the controlled versus natural distinction are repeated in the debates concerning standardized versus criterion-referenced assessment (Lynch & Davidson, 1997) and formal versus informal assessment processes. The processes described by these terms differ to some extent when used in different situations but these different processes can be seen as reflecting the fundamental issues regarding the conditions of sampling. *Standardized* assessments have prescribed protocols for their administration, and these protocols specify the assessment context (usually a clinical setting) and discourse tasks (usually a series of elicitations at word, sentence and sometimes short paragraph levels or in short turn-taking exchanges) and tightly constrain the interactive role of both the assessor (to ask questions, to elicit) and the person being assessed (to respond). Standardized assessments commonly provide normative data on groups of people who are likely to be similar in all other pertinent respects to the person being assessed, and this provision of a reference standard is one of the strongest arguments for their usefulness (Cartwright, 1993). When the person being assessed is different from the normative group in significant ways, however, such as in being from a different country, ethnic culture, subculture, or social class, then the comparison with the reference group raises serious questions regarding the validity of the assessment process for those persons concerned. The developers of standardized tests clearly indicate that such misapplication of test norms is inappropriate, but the lack of available normative data on diverse populations certainly raises the question of how such tests are being used. If the normative reference is not the point of using a standardized test, then such tests may provide a form of description or baseline of performance to enable comparison across a group of persons (for research purposes) or across repeated testing over time (for clinical purposes in the measurement of progress). Using standardized testing in this way provides clinicians with a rudimentary form of criterion-referenced assessment—rudimentary because standardized tests typically do not provide sufficiently detailed hierarchies of levels of achievement. Standardized tests provide too few examples of performance across the range of aspects of communication, and too few examples of performance at each level of performance for each aspect, to render them useful as sufficiently sensitive measures of progress (McCauley & Swisher, 1984). *Criterion-referenced* assessments provide standardized conditions and processes of sampling, and aim to provide greater depth of description of performance, but few such assessments are available, and those that are available suffer from the same limitations just described, in providing limited description of selected aspects of performance with too few examples at each level of performance. In more recent years, cognitive neuropsychological approaches to assessment have harnessed standardized assessment processes to the task of systematically testing a series of hypotheses regarding the integrity of a person's performance in relation to a theoretical conception of the cognitive-linguistic system (Byng, Kay, Edmundson, & Scott, 1990). This focus on the theoretical concepts underlying assessment, rather than the application of normative standards, also has been discussed with regard to child language by Muma (1998).

The dichotomy of formal versus informal assessment also reflects the distinction drawn between controlled and natural sampling. Assessment often is described as *formal* when the process has included standardized testing, and this term also would cover use of a published criterion-referenced assessment tool. Assessment is described as *informal* when it incorporates observational assessment, usually in either natural situations or elicited naturalistic situations. An alternative version of the formal-informal distinction is that of the formal-functional distinction, in which *functional* often is taken to be synonymous with *informal*. This is not, strictly speaking, the case, because formal (as in standardized) assessments of functional language use have been developed, such as the test for "Communicative Activities in Daily Living" (Holland, Frattali, & Fromm, 1998). Functional assessments do focus on natural or naturalistic sampling, however, so they commonly form part of an informal assessment process. Nevertheless, functional assessments too offer varying degrees of naturalness and ecological validity (Worrall, McCooey, Davidson, Larkins, & Hickson, 2002). Informal assessment usually is taken to incorporate discourse sampling, although differing methods are used to analyze the data collected, ranging from online checklists (Prutting & Kirchner, 1987), to checklists based on transcription (Damico, 1985), to linguistic analyses based on transcription (Miller, 1996). Some researchers working with discourse sampling work toward establishing normative references for comparison (Hewitt, Hammer, Yont, & Tomblin, 2005), whereas others have argued for the sample to form an individualized criterion reference point for the client (Armstrong, 2002; Thomson, 2005).

In this chapter, these debates, and some of the issues that flow from them, are deconstructed from a critical discourse perspective. The term *deconstruc-*

tion was coined in the work of Derrida (the leading philosopher in the post-structuralist movement), and although the term carries a negative connotation, he stresses that the process involves understanding how social meanings are "con"-structed with a view to positive improvements (Derrida, 2004; Smith, 2005; Usher, 2000). In speech-language pathology, the use of the term *informal* is intriguing, and deconstruction of the term allows consideration of possible interpretive layers. Derrida's work points out that pairs of terms in binary oppositions do not represent equal social values, and the formal-informal opposition is one in which informal appears to be held as of less value, as, for example, when speech pathology students say, "It was only an informal assessment, but . . . " Informal assessment, even among strong proponents, is seen as requiring some kind of defense, such as suggesting that observational data can be conducted in " . . . an informal, *but systematic* manner" [italics added] (Marquardt & Gillam, 1999, p. 255). In a similar vein, as part of an overview of the assessment of pragmatics, Adams states: "No matter how informal the assessment, if time permits it is always of value to carry out . . . " (Adams, 2002, p. 982).

Some of the problem with the term *informal* arises with the word-level semantics involving a negative rather than a positive meaning. Possibly, the relationship of the word *informal* to other words gives rise to connotations of casual (as in "informal dress" or "informal manner"). By contrast, *formal* connotes proper (in the context of "formal dress," for example) or structured or refined (as in "formal manner"), and perhaps formal assessment processes

pick- up some of this gloss. In speech-language pathology textbooks and reference works, expert authors discuss the importance of informal assessment, making clear and explicit statements about the value of informal assessment, and usually link informal assessment closely with detailed observation in natural environments. Of note, however, formal, standardized assessments typically are dealt with first, before informal assessments are discussed. At the discourse-semantic level, informal assessments are additional (as in "formal *and* informal" assessment) and hence carry the logical but implicit value of being inherently insufficient. Generally speaking, textbooks do not suggest that clinicians need to consider, for example, whether they will conduct a "formal *or* informal" assessment. An exception to this emerges in discussion of the assessment of bilingual persons (Kritikos, 2003), in which the limitations of standardized assessment with regard to validity are recognized, but such discussions are marginal to the broader concern here. The issues are seen as special with regard to this population, despite statistical evidence that bilingualism is the global norm, and despite the relevance of the concerns regarding the need for greater recognition of the inherent limitations of standardized testing.

Of interest, case history taking, which is highly valued in the field and typically is described as occurring first in the sequence of assessment procedures, often is described as separate from other assessments, both formal and informal. In other words, a clear opportunity arises to recognize and describe informal assessment as both the first-indicated assessment component and as the priority in the assessment process—for example, "first conduct an informal assessment (case history, natural-naturalistic observation); then (if needed, for specified purposes) conduct standardized assessment." Nevertheless, informal assessment practices run in second (or, in fact, third) place. Textbooks, of course, are idealized representations, and perhaps in real practice, expert speech-language pathologists in fact follow the informal—then formal approach, but little relevant information is available (Records & Tomblin, 1994). Studies that have attempted to look at assessment practices with regard to outcome measurement have shed some light incidentally on the degree to which standardized tests are seen as useful for the determination of outcomes, and these are discussed later in the chapter (Simmons-Mackie & Damico, 2001).

An important consideration is that the limitations on the uses of standardized assessments have been known and cogently discussed for more than 30 years. Furthermore, methods of informal assessment have been researched widely, with considerable empirical evidence supporting the same type and level of claims to validity as for standardized assessment—for example, the work of Doyle and colleagues in establishing strong psychometric properties for discourse sampling and analysis (Doyle, Goda, & Spencer, 1995; Doyle, Tsironas, Goda, & Kalinyak, 1996; Doyle et al., 1998, 2000; McNeil, Doyle, Fossett, & Park, 2001). Why, then, does much of the relevant literature feature a relative devaluing of informal assessment methods (as indicated by idealized descriptions of the assessment process) and a continued defensive

posture (Duchan, Hewitt, & Sonnenmeier, 1994; Holland, 1991)? Why does experience suggest that even expert practitioners cloak or excuse their reliance on informal assessment? Answers to such questions as these may well lie in the sociopolitical context in which speech-language pathology assessment is framed, rather than resting on the internal debates of relative validity and reliability; this possibility is explored further later on. Similar issues arise in considering not just the process of assessment but also what aspects of communication are assessed; these are discussed next.

Aspects of Communication

The three functions of any act of communication as described in terms of the *metafunctions* of language by Halliday are ideational (experiential-logical), interpersonal, and textual (Halliday & Matthiessen, 2004). Although professionals working from other frameworks may not use these particular terms, other terms such as *transactional* and *interactional* aspects of communication closely shadow these concepts. As discussed in Chapter 1, the pragmatic paradigm that started to influence speech-language pathology during the 1980s raised a number of debates regarding the relative importance of these aspects of communication for understanding the nature of communication disorder and for directing the focus of therapy (Adams, 2002; Prutting, 1982; Prutting & Kirchner, 1983).

First, a pragmatic perspective drew attention to the need to consider interpersonal-interactional aspects of communication as primary, a place previously held by transactional aspects. The focus of most eliciting tasks (controlled or naturalistic) involved consideration of the adequacy of the exchange of information, or the exchange of goods and services in terms of what was said, rather than how the relative interpersonal and social roles of the participants were created or maintained through the interaction. For example, standardized formal tests such as the Western Aphasia Battery (Kertesz, 1982) could indicate what sorts of questions someone with a traumatic brain injury understood, and what information that person could convey in a description of a picture, but it could not describe the person's coherence and turn-taking in interaction, as would, say, the informal observational assessment protocols of Penn (1985) or Prutting and Kirchner (1987). Currently, the focus on transactional and interactional-interpersonal aspects seems fairly equally balanced in the published literature. Clinically, a rather complex relationship between severity of disorder (as perceived by the clinician) and the relative balance of focus for therapy has evolved, such that interactional-interpersonal aspects at the discourse-semantic level are a high priority in working with people with very severe or mild disorders, whereas ideational or transactional

aspects at the lexicogrammatical and discourse-semantic level are a high priority for therapy for such disorders at the moderate range of severity (see Figure 2–1). So, for example, therapy for adults with global aphasia or children with severe autism may focus on turn-taking and use of intonation to signal question versus statement distinctions; therapy for adults with mild aphasia or children with Asperger's syndrome may focus on use of politeness markers; and therapy for adults with moderate aphasia or children with specific language impairment may focus more on noun and verb use to convey information in transitive versus intransitive grammatical sentence structures.

Second, the pragmatic perspective challenged the construct of accuracy as the goal of therapy, arguing for it to be replaced with the construct of adequacy. This debate essentially is about the relative importance of the textual aspects of language, and about deciding upon those textual aspects of language that matter in order to understand the nature of communication disorder, and in order to determine the directions for therapy. At a concrete level, the mode of discourse widened to include nonverbal communication as an aspect to be assessed and treated (whether seen as part of the problem, or as part

Level of Discourse	Ideational Function (Transactional)	Interpersonal Function (Interactional)	Textual Function
Genre			
Discourse-semantic		Severe	
Lexico-grammatical	Moderate		Mild

Figure 2–1. Focus of therapy and severity of communication impairment.

of the potential strategy for compensating for the problem). More recent developments both within the pragmatic perspective and in other sociolinguistic perspectives (including clinical applications of systemic functional linguistics) have seen this argument extended further to a challenge of the deficit focus of speech-language pathology assessment. Instead of using error analyses as the basis for the description of the person's communication and as the basis for determining the targets for therapy, a sociolinguistic perspective argues for the identification of available communication resources as the basis for description and formulation of therapy in both adult neurological caseloads (Armstrong, 1993, 1995; Armstrong, Ferguson, Mortensen, & Togher, 2005) and caseloads involving language learning disability in children (Ruiz, 1995a, 1995b). In other words, textual aspects of language continue to be the major tool for formulating behavioral descriptions of therapy targets, but the focus moves from what clients *cannot* do to what they *can* do.

Both of these issues—which aspect of communication is the focus for therapy and how the disorder is to be judged (that is, in terms of accuracy or adequacy)—give rise to critical questions. What drives decisions about the focus on transactional or interpersonal aspects of communication, and (as has been tentatively suggested) if this balance of focus shifts with severity, what sociocultural assumptions may underlie such choices? What sociocultural frameworks inform the identification of error and the determination of when the presence of error becomes problematic? If deficits and resources can be seen as two parts of the same picture,

then when and how do speech-language pathologists shift their perceptual gestalt so that one and not the other is moved to the foreground or into the background?

Sociocultural Context of Assessment

Thus far it has been argued that the key issues in assessment are influenced by factors outside the internal constructs of validity, and one place to look for the influences on these issues may be in a wider, sociocultural context.

As introduced in Chapter 1, a critical discourse perspective recognizes the way language reflects power relationships in society and at the same time recognizes the way language is used to create power relationships. Power can be seen to operate at three levels: ideological, institutional, and discourse levels. With regard to assessment, *ideological* power encapsulates the culturally accepted views as to what is or is not considered a disorder of communication, and what is seen to be the appropriate way to manage it. So, in Western ideology, standard communication is valued, and deviation from that standard carries negative value (*standard* meaning that which conforms to a common notion regarding what is normal, whether that typically is occurring or not). At the same time, this Western cultural ideology holds that action can, and must, be taken to bring communication toward the standard, and this is summarized in Table 2–1 with reference to culture. *Institutional* power sets up the situation in the community in which tests are required for bureaucratic purposes, for example,

Table 2-1. Discourse Features Associated with Assessment across Personal, Community, and Cultural Contexts

Aspect of Assessment	Discourse Features	Examples	Context		
			Personal	Community (Institutional)	Cultural
Field—topic, agenda, purpose of discourse	*Lexicogrammar*—technical versus lay terminology; transitivity *Discourse-semantics*—reference chains referring to client, clinician, problem	Jargon Passive versus active: "It was found . . . ." "We . . . ."	Display/understand the problem	Recommendation, recognition of need for services	Identification, recognition as problem
Tenor—interpersonal social role/relationship, power, status, distance	*Lexicogrammar*—mood/modality *Discourse-semantics*—role in exchange of information or services (primary, secondary), opportunities for dynamic moves (repair)	Hedging: "It appears that . . ."; ". . . would be recommended"	Constraints on allowable contributions defined by assessment process	Roles and power of clinician and client reflect community values, standards, e.g., qualifications	Culture identifies communication disorder, and assumes it to be remediable
Mode—role of language in the interaction, including channel (verbal, gestural, graphic)	*Lexicogrammar*—linguistic relationship between words (e.g., synonyms) *Discourse-semantics*—theme (highlighted information in first position in clause, paragraph, text)	Synonyms: "disorder"/"difficulty"/ "problem"	Language used to elicit, judge; language as the object of study and the tool for studying it, and the tool for reporting it	Language becomes "data," e.g., transformed by qualitative or quantitative description	Culturally produced taxonomies of communication disorders

such as reporting outcomes of services or providing tools to manage gatekeeping for access to services.

Two main types of *discourse* are used for the purpose of speech-language assessment—the assessment session (see also Chapter 6) and the assessment report. Some of the ways in which the discourse reflects and creates the relative power of those persons involved in the process (see Table 2–1) are discussed next.

The *assessment session* involves most immediately the clinician and the client but also is shaped by the influence of family or caregivers (whether present and actively involved or not) and the referral source. In terms of the *field* of discourse, each participant brings a different agenda to the situation, which has an impact on the discourse. Congruent agenda can be seen when the clinician seeks to understand the problem through successive and systematic elicitations and the client seeks to display the problem through responsive contributions. However, when the client seeks to understand the problem (for example, through asking questions, seeking clarification) during the constrained context of standardized testing elicitation, then the *tenor* of the discourse is affected, as the interpersonal role relationship between the clinician and the client alters through this discoursal shift. Informal assessment processes potentially allow more opportunity for clients to exert power in the relationship, and fewer constraints in the observation and sampling process allow for more flexibility in the turn-taking exchange and opportunities for repair. Also, clients can draw the clinician's attention to aspects of the discourse that they find particu-

larly troublesome, for example. The power relationship within the session is complex, in that the clinician "serves" the client, so the client holds the power to request or refuse services, while at the same time within the session, the clinician takes the powerful role of initiating, leading, and ending the discourse.

The *assessment report* moves the personal experience into the community context, in that the purpose of the report is to make recommendations regarding services. The role of the clinician is prescribed by community expectations and standards, with the report explicitly stating the position of the speech-language pathologist in the organization, and their community-recognized qualifications. Textually, the discourse observed during the assessment process becomes transformed into data, so that language behaviors become percentages, and so on. As analyzed from a critical discourse perspective by Duchan, assessment reports take the form of a particular genre with a highly predictable macrostructure (presentations, observations, conclusions, recommendations), and analysis of their content reveals a problem focus that situates the client as the owner of the problem and frames the speech-language pathologist as the solution (Duchan, 1999). Generally speaking, assessment reports use lengthy reference chains involving the client, while at the same time removing the clinician as active agent, through the use of passive and existential constructions ("*it was* found . . . "). The power of the conclusions drawn is laid out as negotiable through the use of modalization (hedging) ("it *would* appear that . . . "). These two discourse strategies are ways in which the clinician seeks to conform to professional community standards of objectivity, explicitly seen as a valued property of assessment reports. The third strategy for enhancing the objectivity of reports is through the provision of behavioral description, yet the clinician has made subjective judgments regarding which behaviors are salient and thus which behaviors are to be reported. Essentially, an assessment report can be seen as an opinion in which the power of the clinician to judge is masked discoursally.

One of the major sociocultural influences on assessment and intervention practices relates to the high social value placed on science during the span of the development of the speech-language pathology profession (Apel, 1999; Siegel, 1987; Siegel & Ingham, 1987). In other areas, such as medicine, a shift from religion to science has occurred as the socially valued source of theory and practice, and certainly some of the more medical aspects of speech-language pathology have seen similar shifts. The discipline of speech-language pathology, however, emerged in the twentieth century, along with related disciplines such as psychology, at a time when the scientific paradigm became dominant. Although arguably all modern science is relatively new (arising in the past century or so), speech-language pathology is both newer (arising after World War II in identified training programs) and somewhat precariously placed with respect to just how "scientific" it is (Ringel, Trachtman, & Prutting, 1984). In common with other disciplines whose reason for being is the provision of education and therapy, speech-language pathology contains another binary opposition with cultural signif-

icance—art versus science. This dichotomy provides competing paradigms that inform theory and practice. The *art* of speech-language pathology (that is, the creative and interpretive processes involved) may be discussed in professional development activities, conference papers, and non–peer-reviewed papers, but it is the *science* (that is, the analytical processes) that has higher social value both inside and outside the discipline, as indicated by dissemination in peer-reviewed journals. In a cultural framework in which science has high status, controlled sampling in laboratory-like conditions is more "scientific," despite the evidence of equivalent rigor obtainable through naturalistic sampling, and despite the evidence of what Cicourel describes as "white room effects" that contaminate validity (Cicourel, 1996). Of note, such "white room effects" are not just associated with laboratory or clinical conditions but may be observed in more naturalistic research—for example, in ethnographic studies, where the field notes become the data and so are abstracted from the events themselves.

The previously discussed debates in the profession about methods of sampling, and aspects of communication to be sampled, are conducted within an analytical, empirical, science-based perspective (Baker & Chenery, 1997) and therefore reflect the modern, *positivist* perspective. Both sides of these debates (whether for or against control, or for particular aspects of communication as central) assume the existence of a "right" method that can identify the real nature of the disorder. As previously mentioned, sociopolitical power is evidenced in that the high social status of science confers privilege to controlled, standardized assessment of transactional aspects of communication in which the focus of assessment is on the identification of errors as defined in comparison with a normative reference group. This "privileging" process underpins the use of this assessment methodology in clinical situations in which the test developers themselves would deem such use inappropriate and prompts clinicians to provide defensive justification when their assessment decision-making processes lead them to choose the less privileged option, to devalue the information gained thereby, and (consciously or unconsciously) to fail to recognize or acknowledge when they are using these options.

In research on expert and novice workers whose duties and tasks involved identifying customer needs and negotiating products and prices (Laufer & Glick, 1996), it was suggested that novices tended to "toe the company line" in following rules and required procedures, whereas experts strategically and creatively adapted procedures with an end-goal focus. It is likely that expert speech-language pathologists routinely shift the balance of their assessment methods to suit the end-goal (possibly their own end-goals, such as a time-efficient assessment, and optimally their clients' end-goals, such as an assessment of their priority needs for therapy). This process of clinical decision-making remains implicit, however, so presumably experts fail to reflect on their own practice and novices must pick up such unexamined practices osmotically.

An alternative to a positivist perspective is an *interpretive*, or *postpositivist*, perspective, in which it is acknowl-edged that different interpretations are possible and not necessarily mutually exclusive. From an interpretive perspective, full understanding of the nature of communication is not possible, but useful insights can be gained into its nature through different perspectives and interpretations. The emphasis here is on usefulness, in that interpretive thinking (from a Habermas viewpoint) is one in which interpretations are judged not for their "rightness" but with reference to their utility for the problem at hand. The recognition of the importance of multiple perspectives is consistent with the needs of clinical decision-making and in fact is evidenced in diverse frameworks applied to speech-language pathology, including psycholinguistic assessments that stress the need for multiple sources of information (Aram, Morris, & Hall, 1993; Lahey, 1990), and sociolinguistic qualitative assessments that use the term *triangulation* to describe the process by which multiple perspectives inform a description or an interpretation (Damico & Simmons-Mackie, 2003). This process of triangulation is considered next.

Triangulation: Solution or Part of the Problem?

Triangulation as a term is essentially a metaphor loosely borrowed from navigation in which a location can be determined with reference to a map by taking sightings from at least two landmarks. Although this concept of triangulation is very much associated with the qualitative research paradigm, as noted earlier, the use of systematic comparisons from multiple sources of information is common across both positivist and postpositivist perspectives. Accordingly, the following discussion ranges across both perspectives when appropriate. Triangulation can be used to refer to counterpointing information derived from different data, different researchers, different methods, and different theories or disciplines. In clinical decision-making, the practice of obtaining information from multiple sources (e.g., parent, caregiver, teacher), from multiple observations (e.g., clinical, home, or work or school settings), and using multiple methods (e.g., informal or formal assessments) reflects the same general principle. The purpose of such comparison is to look for similarities or differences that would support or refute theory building or hypothesis testing.

Generally speaking, triangulation is held to be evidence of sound methodology through the reduction of bias, and to add to the validity and rigor of research and clinical decision-making. Nevertheless, triangulation is open to criticism on two counts. First, at a practical level, little to no discussion or guidelines have emerged regarding how the comparative process of contrasting information from multiple sources should be carried out (Farmer, Robinson, Elliott, & Eyles, 2006). Can data or findings from methodologically dissimilar projects in fact be validly compared? For example, does the information gained from the Psycholinguistic Assessments of Language Processing (Kay, Lesser, & Coltheart, 1992) relate in any way to information gained from the test for Communicative Abilities in Daily Living (Holland et al., 1998), or do such assessments yield entirely separate data sets? Of greater significance, can analyses and interpretations drawn from fundamentally different perspectives (e.g., quantitative, qualitative) be seen as providing complementary perspectives, or are they alternative perspectives? What weight is attached to the view of the person with the communication problem, and how does this view compete against contrary perspectives? Second, and of greater theoretical significance, if all of the points of comparison are held to provide interpretations of equal value, then how does the researcher or clinician weigh which data are correct, which interpretation is right (if working from a positivist perspective), or which interpretation is the most useful for the present purposes (if working from a postpositivist perspective)? Arguably, triangulation simply introduces additional sources of bias, rather than resolving or neutralizing bias, as discussed by Blaikie (1991, p. 123), who suggests that from a positivist perspective, congruence in measures or findings would suggest a lack of bias and lack of congruence would suggest the possibility of bias, whereas from a postpositivist perspective, congruence would suggest a shared view of the world and lack of congruence may suggest different but valid views of the world (Blaikie, 1991). As Blaikie also suggests, extending the navigational metaphor, the compounding of multiple sources of information and interpretation may leave us " . . . trying to navigate in a fog" (p. 126).

Agnew and colleagues look to find a way through this infinite interpretive dilemma by recognizing that, philosophies of thinking aside, reality exists, although only partial glimpses of it may be possible (Agnew, Ford, & Hayes, 1997). These researchers suggest that the hallmark of an expert is deliberate seeking of not just positives and negatives (that is, identification of problems through convergence of data or refutation of problems through divergence of information) but also active attempts to identify methods that will allow for detection of false positives and false negatives (for example, through obtaining follow-up data checking that identified problems are not later refuted, or determining whether clients initially assessed as not showing problems are not later identified as having such problems). Research projects, of course, often build in this kind of follow-up— but in routine clinical practice, both false positives and false negatives typically are identified in an ad hoc manner (e.g., dependent on assertiveness in requesting review from the same clinical service), rather than through built-in systems associated with assessment processes. Although acknowledging the cultural domination of science inherent in this suggestion, these researchers argue for a kind of knowing, critical acceptance of this cultural influence. They suggest that this approach reflects an expert means-to-an-end strategy aimed at reducing doubt, rather than establishing "truth" (Agnew et al.).

Experts and Triangulation

Speech-language pathology has well-accepted and well-developed methods of making use of different sources of information within the positivist perspective. For example, in both research and clinical work, the establishment of interrater and intrarater agreement is widespread practice (Damico, Oller, & Tetnowski, 1999; O'Brian, O'Brian, Packman, & Onslow, 2003). Speech-language pathologists frequently combine assessment methodologies drawn from widely disparate theoretical models, although whether this practice reflects an informed and considered triangulation is uncertain (Thomson, 2003). Little is known, however, about how speech-language pathologists integrate multiple sources of information for the purposes of clinical decision-making, and about what influences their decision-making (Kamhi, 1994). Blau and colleagues present a brief description of an attempt to look at these issues in their comparison of information gained from standardized language assessment and spontaneous language samples for 10 children in terms of the effect of sampling on the formulation of goals (Blau, Lahey, & Oleksiuk-Velez, 1984). These researchers noted that the standardized test errors were not considered suitable for intervention because they fell outside the next expected developmental sequence for the cases studied, whereas the language sample " . . . led to more specific goals, providing both content and context in which goals should be taught" (Blau et al., p. 79). Insufficient detail regarding how this decision-making occurred was provided, however, to allow greater insight into the processes involved. Records and Tomblin (1994) attempted to look at clinical decision-making by 27 speech-language pathologists who were presented with 92 sets of quantitative test data and asked to determine the presence of language impairment. Records and Tomblin's discussion equates clinical with inferential decision-making, and distinguishes this entity from statistical and quantitative decision-making; because only quantitative data were provided to the speech-language pathologists, it appears that this latter approach was viewed as of higher value. These investigators found that nearly all clinicians made use of comprehension and production data, but that nonverbal intelligence quotient (IQ) data were used variously. The investigators note that these findings might have been different if the speech-language pathologists had access to spontaneous language samples (Records & Tomblin, p. 152). Unfortunately, of the 92 sets of data, 50 (65%) were fabricated (computer-generated) cases, and the extent to which these profile patterns would represent those that expert speech-language pathologists would recognize from the real world is not known. Also, the quantitative data provided subtests abstracted from standardized test profiles, so again, the expert speech-language pathologists did not have access to the types of patterned data that perhaps would be expected in real-world practice.[1]

Roulstone, on the other hand, used a qualitative methodology based on interviews, case analyses and focus group discussions with 11 speech-language pathologists to derive a description of the patterns of decision-making used in the initial assessment of preschool-aged children (described using systemic network depiction drawn from the systemic functional linguistics model) (Roulstone, 1997). The patterns identified indicated a strong reliance on information from communication history, suggesting the importance of this informal aspect of assessment. Throughout the assessment process, potential targets for therapy were being formulated; these possibilities were affecting areas for assessment, suggesting that an end-goal strategy was being used by these clinicians.

Hagstrom (2001) presents a model of decision-making that she proposes would provide an explicit linkage between theory and clinical decision-making. This model sets out six lines of inquiry and reflection (the knowledge domain, the extent of active involvement of the client, the stages involved, the end-goal, the assumed process by which change will occur, the methods for collecting data and documenting change). As noted by Hagstrom, the extent to which clinicians use the aspects of such a model or how they integrate these lines of clinical reasoning has not been investigated. Further research into clinical decision-making practice could build on the lessons learned from such preliminary research into an important issue.

On the basis of novice versus expert research in other fields, it is possible to speculate that although novice speech-language pathologists may collect different sets of data, they may be likely to work within each data set, rather than integrating information (for example, using one particular test for initial assessment, but then making subsequent decisions for therapy based on informal assessment). Expert speech-language pathologists may be more

---

[1]"Perhaps" because research by McAuley and Demetras found in a survey of 72 research studies published between 1983 to 1988 in the area of child language impairment that use of incomplete tests was widespread (McCauley & Demetras, 1990).

likely to recognize complex patterns of client presentation based on initial informal assessment, selecting formal assessment strategies, for example, only when required for particular purposes (funding support for clients, perhaps). From research on everyday expert decision-making in other fields (Laufer & Glick, 1996), it might be hypothesized that part of the pattern that expert speech-language pathologists recognize would be the wider community and cultural factors that will influence directions for intervention likely to be most acceptable and productive for the individual client. Evidence to support such contentions awaits further research, but in the interim, it probably is safe to assume that speech-language pathologists' decision-making with regard to assessment is affected by two movements in both health and education fields: (1) evidence-based practice and (2) accountability as established through reported outcome measures. These two aspects of the current sociocultural climate are considered next.

Evidence-Based Practice and the Assessment of Outcomes

Evidence-based practice and outcomes assessment are interrelated notions, yet they operate in distinctly different ways. *Evidence-based practice* represents a synthesis and application of the best level of research available regarding the efficacy of a particular approach, most usually with respect to intervention but equally applicable to assessment approaches. Evidence-based practice is

strongly influenced by positivist perspectives, in that the "best" is assumed to reflect the extent to which the research is grounded within scientific method. In order to obtain the controls required by scientific method, such research is necessarily different from real-world service settings (for example, research subject selection may be more selective, excluding subjects with previous histories of treatment, and so on). Some critical reviews of evidence-based practice have emerged over time (Drake, Latimer, Leff, McHugo, & Burns, 2004), and attempts have been made to incorporate levels of qualitative rigor within the levels of evidence (Mays, Pope, & Popay, 2005). In idealized statements of day-to-day clinical practice, however, the prevailing social value strongly endorses quantitative methodologies and the scientific method to guide clinical decision-making.

Outcome measures, on the other hand, represent an assessment of the ability of a particular service (which ideally represents an application of evidence-based practice within a real-world setting) to achieve its goals (Frattali, 1998). Determination of outcomes may share features with research (for example, the need for reliability of measurement), but in order to capture the real-world setting, considerable control generally is lost, and measures typically are of broader end-point goals, rather than the more fine-grained research goals. A survey of Australian speech-language pathologists working with child and adult caseloads found that 50% of 249 facilities were using outcome measures, and it appeared that the impetus for their use was driven by the clinicians themselves, rather than by institutional demand (Worrall & Egan, 2001).

As indicated by the work of Simmons and colleagues in the area of aphasia, speech-language pathologists appear to be caught in a paradigm bind in their use of outcome measures between making use of available comprehensive standardized tests and the use of more general descriptive measurement tools (Simmons-Mackie, Threats, & Kagan, 2005). Substantially more standardized assessments designed as linguistic or cognitive measures (127 reports), such as the Boston Diagnostic Aphasia Examination (Goodglass & Kaplan, 1983), were reported as being used, in comparison with reported use of outcome measures (73 reports) such as the American Speech-Language-Hearing Association's (ASHA) Functional Assessment of Communication Skills (FACS) (Frattali, Thompson, Holland, Wohl, & Ferketic, 1995) or Therapy Outcome Measures (Enderby & John, 1997).

Discourse measures have been put forward by many workers as offering potential usefulness as outcome measures. For example, just as percent of syllables stuttered and ratings of severity and naturalness offer quantification that appears to capture important qualitative change in response to stuttering treatment (Onslow & Ingham, 1987), so too do words per minute and ratings of communicative workload appear to capture quantitatively aspects of production that may be sensitive to qualitatively significant changes for adults with aphasia (Ferguson, 1996; Nicholas & Brookshire, 1993). Such quantification, however, represents a substantial distortion of the nature of the aspects of communication with which speech-language pathologists are concerned but also fails to engage with the fundamental goals of therapy, that is, the

achievement of specified changes that have significant impact on the life of the person with communication difficulty. For example, in working with children with specific language impairment, short-term goals may be realized in terms of achieving some particular percentage increase on particular language behaviors, but the more substantive aim may be to increase these children's success in their social and academic worlds (Clegg, Hollis, Mawhood, & Rutter, 2005). In working with adults with acquired aphasia, a short-term goal may be identified as achieving a greater percentage of words retrieved, but the broader aim may be to increase successful participation of these clients in their social and vocational worlds (Hinckley, 2002). The determination of outcomes, with its built-in necessity of incorporating real-world complexity, offers an opportunity to tackle the development of qualitative holistic descriptions of significant aspects of change associated with speech-language pathology interventions.

What is decided on as the system of measures or descriptors of the outcomes of intervention has fundamental importance as a shaper of what is done in therapy. The formulation of therapy goals commonly is described in terms of a forward-planning process based on assessment data. As has been discussed previously in this chapter and in the literature, however, standardized tests provide insufficient information to assist, criterion-referenced tests are not available for most purposes, and informal assessment processes typically are underspecified for this purpose. In actual practice, expert speech-language pathologists instead may determine their end-goals and then work back from that point in developing interventions (Kagan et al., 2003). Such a notion is consistent with the previously discussed research by Laufer and Glick (1996) on expert decision-making that suggested application of this backward formulation strategy in real-world situations, in contrast with previous research in the area.

What is crucially important in adopting such a strategy is consistency between the nature of the goal itself and the determination of the extent to which that end-goal is reached. In the field of education, particularly in the area of foreign language teaching, a much-discussed phenomenon is that of *washback*. Washback refers to that part of the overall impact of a test that is affecting the curriculum or the manner of teaching (Wall, 1997). Washback can be seen to be positive when testing drives learning in ways that benefit learners, but negative when testing results in "teaching to the test" or when the uses to which the test is put result in inequitable consequences for the learner (for example, when used as selection criterion in situations in which the test content is unrelated to the purpose of selection) (Shohamy, 1998, 2001a, 2001b, 2004). Certainly, one of the potential misuses of tests in speech-language pathology is the potential for therapy to be directed toward similar tasks to those contained in the test (rather than using the test to direct further probes and individualized assessment toward therapy formulation). One of the strongest examples within speech-language pathology of the potential inequities associated with testing is in the area of language learning disability, in which tests form part of the gate-keeping function for

access to services such as additional instruction by support teachers or special classroom placement (Lahey, 1990). Diagnostic labels such as "specific language impairment" carry political weight in lobbying for services, but considerable debates surrounds the criteria for their application. Aram and colleagues, in their empirically based comparison of the use of operational criteria in research on specific language impairment and clinical determinations, found a 60% concordance, at best, between the two approaches (Aram et al., 1993). Of interest, these researchers note the high face validity associated with the apparent weight given to parent report in clinical determinations, and they argue strongly against operational criteria as the sole mechanism for diagnosis and service provision. Workers in the education field have recognized the need for development of systematic ways to guide interpretation of test results so that test use is consistent with test design (Bachman, 2005). In speech-language pathology, although experts call for the recognition of the limitations of standardized testing in such situations in the strongest terms (ASHA, 1989, 2000, 2004), clinical decision-making will involve the speech-language pathologist in making recommendations based on a complex synthesis of multiple sources of information and interpretations (as discussed previously). When special placement becomes the end-goal of an assessment, ethical decision-making starts at the point of choosing what to test and how.

In relation to intervention, if tests or outcome measures are selected that do not reflect the end-goals, then it should not be a surprise when little or insignificant changes are seen to occur in these measures after therapy. For example, in developing group therapy for people with chronic aphasia aiming to improve psychosocial function, determination of outcome through such tools as the Visual Analogue Self-Esteem Scale (Brumfitt & Sheeran, 1999) may be more appropriate than psycholinguistic measures (Alston, Sherratt, Ferguson, & Vajak, 2006). Determination of end-goals, however, also is a socially situated process. Earlier in this chapter, it was suggested that speech-language pathologists made decisions regarding the focus of therapy (ideational-transactional, interpersonal, textual) that were influenced largely by severity. This possibility opens wider social questions: For example, when severity is factored into decision-making, does the likely efficacy of specific approaches with persons with communication disorders at particular severity levels enter into decisions regarding the type and availability of services? Certainly, some evidence exists that would move decision-making in this direction. A speech-language pathologist may be reasonably confident, for example, that for a person with global aphasia, the end-goal for verbal production will be short of complete sentences, and this recognition may prompt a decision to focus on the use of augmentative modes of communication for the mediation of interpersonal exchanges. In speech-language pathology, however, strong evidence more often is lacking than present, and clinicians deal with individual responses to therapy, not with average responses as reported in larger-scale research. Some ways forward in this situation have been suggested from the positivist perspective through the

adoption of within-subject experimental designs as a framework for intervention (Franklin, Allison, & Gorman, 1997; Thompson, 2006), and from perspectives that are more along postpositivist lines in their prioritorization of participant perspectives—for example, the collaborative development of end-goals with persons with communication disorders (Worrall, 2006), such as through use of tools such as the Functional Communication Therapy Planner (Worrall, 1999).

All of the ways described for the assessment decision-making process, however, fail to take into account the wider sociopolitical context in which the speech-language pathologist practices. Speech-language pathologists working in a range of situations will no doubt recognize the situation in which they are encouraged by their employing body to participate in evidence-based practice professional development activities, while at the same time having proposals rejected for the additional funding for the staff and resources required to deliver evidence-based treatment (such as intensive aphasia therapy). Possibly one of the biggest contributors to clinician burnout is the point at which speech-language pathologists become aware that their clinical decisions inevitably will be constrained by the institutional and wider cultural contexts in which they are working. Although some discussion is ongoing regarding such situations in terms of clashes between the speech-pathologist's personal and professional values and those of the institution (Byng, Cairns, & Duchan, 2002; Worrall, 2000), the tendency is to internalize this debate (in the sense of seeing this as a problem to be "owned" by speech-language pathologists), rather than recognizing the wider social context (Byng & Duchan, 2005). With this kind of dissonance between personal and social values, the risk of losing experts in the profession increases, or experts who remain in practice may become disillusioned and strategic, rather than client-focused. Alternatively, in line with the focus of this book, experts may become critically focused and develop ways to promote change.

Future Directions

So how, then, to proceed from a critical perspective? First, it has been argued that the recurring debates within speech-language pathology regarding the validity claims of differing methods of assessment need to be recognized as offering different interpretations of the nature of communication, rather than particular approaches representing a more or less accurate reflection of communication. It is insufficient for most clinical purposes, however, to hold multiple interpretations in a simultaneous prismatic reflection, as suggested by Wolfram Cox from a business management perspective (Wolfram Cox, 1999), when the task is to solve particular problems in working with people on an individual basis. Because speech-language pathologists, novice and expert alike, are integrating such diverse perspectives on a daily basis, a useful direction for further consideration within a critical perspective is the investigation of how they are achieving this everyday problem-solving within their interpersonal, institutional, and wider cultural contexts.

Second, it has been suggested that the relationship between assessment and intervention probably is not simply unidirectional, in that assessment drives intervention (and indeed that direction has been queried as potentially negative for clients). Instead, the relationship has been suggested to be bidirectional, in that end-goals (with currently unclear derivation associated with social and political influences) drive intervention and the selection of measures of outcome. A greater understanding of the rationales for the determination of therapy is needed (Worrall, 2006; Worrall et al., 2006) in order to consider how decisions are made, as well as to provide explicit guidance for novice speech-language pathologists.

Third, in this chapter it has been suggested that assessment arises from and serves sociopolitical purposes, as can be seen in today's outcomes assessment approach and evidence-based practice. It is suggested that speech-language pathologists in their role of assessors share the social responsibility, as discussed by Shohamy (2001) with regard to educational language testers, not just for the development of appropriate assessments but also for constant vigilance and activism with regard to their equitable use. At an immediate and local level, speech-language pathologists (particularly those with the institutional power associated with seniority and expertise) need to consider the assessment practices to which their professional services are contributing. In the longer term, further investigation of the uses and abuses of testing in speech-language pathology warrants attention.

In the next chapter, the focus on assessment is continued, in order to examine more closely the dynamic aspects of the integrative processes involved in assessment.

References

Adams, C. (2002). Practitioner review: The assessment of language pragmatics. *Journal of Child Psychology & Psychiatry, 43*(8), 973–987.

Agnew, N. M., Ford, K. M., & Hayes, P. J. (1997). Expertise in context: Personally constructed, socially selected and reality-relevant? In P. J. Feltovich, K. M. Ford, & R. R. Hoffman (Eds.), *Expertise in context: Human and machine* (pp. 220–244). Menlo Park, CA: AAAI Press/MIT Press.

Alston, M., Sherratt, S., Ferguson, A., & Vajak, J. (2006). *Outcomes in a chronic aphasia group: Measures and results.* Paper presented at the "Stroke: It's time" 2nd Australasian Nursing and Allied Health Stroke Conference, Sydney, July 6–7.

American Speech-Language-Hearing Association. (1989, March). Issues in determining eligibility for language intervention. *American Speech-Language-Hearing Association's Committee on Language Learning Disorders,* 113–118.

American Speech-Language-Hearing Association. (2000). *IDEA and your caseload: A template for eligibility and dismissal criteria for students aged 3 to 21.* Rockville, MD: Author.

American Speech-Language-Hearing Association. (2004). Admission/discharge criteria in speech-language pathology. *ASHA Supplement, 24,* 65–70.

Apel, K. (1999). Checks and balances: Keeping the science in our profession. *Language, Speech, and Hearing Services in Schools, 30*(1), 98–107.

Aram, D. M., Morris, R., & Hall, N. E. (1993). Clinical and research congruence in identifying children with specific language impairment. *Journal of Speech & Hearing Research, 36,* 580–591.

Armstrong, E. (1993). Aphasia rehabilitation: A sociolinguistic perspective. In A. J. Holland & M. M. Forbes (Eds.), *Aphasia treatment: World perspectives* (pp. 263–290). San Diego, CA: Singular.

Armstrong, E. (1995). A linguistic approach to the functional skills of aphasic speakers. In C. Code & D. Muller (Eds.), *Treatment of aphasia: From theory to practice* (pp. 70–89). London: Whurr.

Armstrong, E. (2002). Variation in the discourse of non–brain-damaged speakers on a clinical task. *Aphasiology, 16*(4/5/6), 647–658.

Armstrong, E., Ferguson, A., Mortensen, L., & Togher, L. (2005). Acquired language disorders: Some functional insights. In R. Hasan, J. Webster, & C. Matthiessen (Eds.), *Continuing discourse on language* (Vol. 1). London: Equinox.

Bachman, L. R. (2005). Building and supporting a case for test use. *Language Assessment Quarterly, 2*(1), 1–34.

Baker, R., & Chenery, H. (1997). The assessment of speech and language disorders. In C. Clapham & D. Corson (Eds.), *Encyclopedia of language and education: Language testing and assessment* (Vol. 7, pp. 211–233). Dordrecht: Kluwer.

Banerjee, J., & Luoma, S. (1997). Qualitative approaches to test validation. In C. Clapham & D. Corson (Eds.), *Encyclopedia of language and education: Language testing and assessment* (Vol. 7, pp. 275–287). Dordrecht: Kluwer.

Blaikie, N. W. H. (1991). A critique of the use of triangulation in social research. *Quality & Quantity, 25,* 115–136.

Blau, A. F., Lahey, M., & Oleksiuk-Velez, A. (1984). Planning goals for intervention: Language testing or language sampling? *Exceptional Children, 51*(1), 78–79.

Bornstein, M. H., Painter, K. M., & Park, J. (2002). Naturalistic language sampling in typically developing children. *Journal of Child Language, 29,* 687–699.

Brumfitt, S., & Sheeran, P. (1999). *VASES: Visual analogue self-esteem scale.* Bicester, UK: Winslow.

Byng, S., Cairns, D., & Duchan, J. (2002). Values in practice and practising values. *Journal of Communication Disorders, 35*, 89–106.

Byng, S., & Duchan, J. F. (2005). Social model philosophies and principles: Their applications to therapies for aphasia. *Aphasiology, 19*(10/11), 906–922.

Byng, S., Kay, J., Edmundson, A., & Scott, C. M. (1990). Aphasia tests reconsidered. *Aphasiology, 4*(1), 67–91.

Cartwright, L. R. (1993). The challenge of interpreting test scores. *Clinics in Communication Disorders, 3*(3), 17–25.

Chaytor, N., & Schmitter-Edgecombe, M. (2003). The ecological validity of neuropsychological tests: A review of the literature on everyday cognitive skills. *Neuropsychology Review, 13*(4), 181–197.

Cicourel, A. V. (1996). Ecological validity and 'white room effects': The interaction of cognitive and cultural models in the pragmatic analysis of elicited narratives from children. *Pragmatics & Cognition, 4*(2), 221–264.

Clegg, J., Hollis, C., Mawhood, L., & Rutter, M. (2005). Developmental language disorders—a follow-up in later adult life. Cognitive, language and psychosocial outcomes. *Journal of Child Psychology & Psychiatry, 46*(2), 128–149.

Damico, J. S. (1985). Clinical discourse analysis: A functional approach to language assessment. In C. S. Simon (Ed.), *Communication skills and classroom success: Assessment of language learning disabled students.* San Diego, CA: College-Hill.

Damico, J. S., Oller, J. W., & Tetnowski, J. A. (1999). Investigating the interobserver reliability of a direct observational language assessment technique. *Advances in Speech Language Pathology, 1*(2), 77–94.

Damico, J. S., & Simmons-Mackie, N. (2003). Qualitative research and speech-language pathology: A tutorial for the clinical realm. *American Journal of Speech-Language Pathology, 12*(2), 131–143.

Derrida, J. (2004). *Positions* (A. Bass, Trans.) [Originally published in France in 1972 as *Positions* by Les Editions de Minuit.]. London: Continuum.

Doyle, P. J., Goda, A. J., & Spencer, K. A. (1995). The communicative informativeness and efficiency of connected discourse by adults with aphasia under structured and conversational sampling conditions. *American Journal of Speech-Language Pathology, 4*, 130–134.

Doyle, P. J., McNeil, M. R., Park, G., Goda, A., Rubenstein, E., Spencer, K., et al. (2000). Linguistic validation of four parallel forms of a story retelling procedure. *Aphasiology, 14*, 537–549.

Doyle, P. J., McNeil, M. R., Spencer, K. A., Goda, A. J., Cottrell, K., & Lustig, A. (1998). The effects of concurrent picture presentation on retelling of orally-presented stories by adults with aphasia. *Aphasiology, 12*, 561–573.

Doyle, P. J., Tsironas, D., Goda, A. J., & Kalinyak, M. (1996). The relationship between objective measures and listener's judgements of communicative informativeness of the connected discourse of adults with aphasia. *American Journal of Speech-Language Pathology, 5*, 53–60.

Drake, R. E., Latimer, E. A., Leff, H. S., McHugo, G. J., & Burns, B. J. (2004). What is evidence? *Child and Adolescent Psychiatric Clinics of North America, 13*, 717–728.

Duchan, J. F. (1999). Reports written by speech-language pathologists: The role of agenda in constructing client competence. In D. Kovarsky, J. F. Duchan, & M. Maxwell (Eds.), *Constructing (in)competence: Disabling evaluations in clinical and social interaction* (pp. 223–224). Mahwah, NJ: Lawrence Erlbaum Associates.

Duchan, J. F., Hewitt, L. E., & Sonnenmeier, R. M. (1994). Three themes: Stage two pragmatics, combating marginalization, and the relation of theory and practice. In J. F. Duchan, L. E. Hewitt, & R. M. Sonnenmeier (Eds.), *Pragmatics: From theory to practice* (pp. 1–9). Englewood Cliffs, NJ: Prentice-Hall.

Enderby, P., & John, A. (1997). *Therapy outcome measures: Speech-language pathology.* San Diego, CA: Singular.

Farmer, T., Robinson, K., Elliott, S. J., & Eyles, J. (2006). Developing and implementing a triangulation protocol for qualitative health research. *Qualitative Health Research, 16*(3), 377–394.

Ferguson, A. (1996). Describing competence in aphasic/normal conversation. *Clinical Linguistics & Phonetics, 10*(1), 55–63.

Franklin, R. D., Allison, D. B., & Gorman, B. S. (Eds.). (1997). *Design and analysis of single-case research.* Mahwah, NJ: Lawrence Erlbaum Associates.

Frattali, C. (Ed.). (1998). *Measuring outcomes in speech-language pathology.* New York: Thieme.

Frattali, C. M., Thompson, C. K., Holland, A. L., Wohl, C. B., & Ferketic, M. M. (1995). *Functional assessment of communication skills for adults (FACS).* Rockville, MD: American Speech-Language-Hearing Association.

Goodglass, H., & Kaplan, E. (1983). *Boston diagnostic examination for aphasia.* Philadelphia: Lea & Febiger.

Habermas, J. (1972). *Knowledge and human interests* (J. J. Shapiro, Trans.). London: Heinemann Educational.

Hagstrom, F. (2001). Using and building theory in clinical action. *Journal of Communication Disorders, 34,* 371–384.

Halliday, M. A. K., & Matthiessen, C. M. I. M. (2004). *An introduction to functional grammar* (3rd ed.). London: Arnold.

Hewitt, L. E., Hammer, C. S., Yont, K. M., & Tomblin, J. B. (2005). Language sampling for kindergarten children with and without SLI: Mean length of utterance, IPSYN, and NDW. *Journal of Communication Disorders, 38,* 197–213.

Hinckley, J. J. (2002). Vocational and social outcomes of adults with chronic aphasia. *Journal of Communication Disorders, 35*(6), 543–560.

Holland, A. L. (1991). Pragmatic aspects of intervention in aphasia. *Journal of Neurolinguistics, 6*(2), 197–211.

Holland, A. L., Frattali, C., & Fromm, D. (1998). *Communication activities of daily living* (2nd ed.). Austin, TX: Pro-Ed.

Kagan, A., Simmons-Mackie, N., & Threats, T. T. (2003). *Beginning with the end: Participation-based outcome evaluation in aphasia.* Paper presented at the American Speech-Language-Hearing Association Convention, Chicago.

Kamhi, A. G. (1994, April). Toward a theory of clinical expertise in speech-language pathology. *Language, Speech, and Hearing Services in Schools, 25,* 115–118.

Kay, J., Lesser, R., & Coltheart, M. (1992). *Psycholinguistic assessment of language processing in aphasia (PALPA).* Hove, East Sussex, England: Lawrence Erlbaum.

Kazdin, A. E. (2003). *Research design in clinical psychology.* Boston: Allyn & Bacon.

Kertesz, A. (1982). *The western aphasia battery.* New York: Grune & Stratton.

Kritikos, E. P. (2003). Speech-language pathologists' beliefs about language assessment of bilingual/bicultural individuals. *American Journal of Speech-Language Pathology, 12*(1), 73–91.

Lahey, M. (1990). Who shall be called language disordered? Some reflections and one perspective. *Journal of Speech & Hearing Disorders, 55,* 612–620.

Laufer, E. A., & Glick, J. (1996). Expert and novice differences in cognition and activity: A practical work activity. In Y. Engestrom & D. Middleton (Eds.), *Cognition and communication at work* (pp. 177–198). Cambridge: Cambridge University Press.

Lynch, B. K., & Davidson, F. (1997). Criterion referenced testing. In C. Clapham & D. Corson (Eds.), *Encyclopedia of language and education: Language testing and assessment* (Vol. 7, pp. 263–273). Dordrecht: Kluwer.

Marquardt, T. P., & Gillam, R. B. (1999). Assessment in communication disorders: Some observations on current issues. *Language Testing, 16*(3), 249–269.

Mays, N., Pope, C., & Popay, J. (2005). Systematically reviewing qualitative and quantitative evidence to inform management and policy-making in the health field. *Journal of Health Services Research & Policy, 10*(Suppl. 1), S6–S20.

McCauley, R. J., & Demetras, M. J. (1990). The identification of language impairment in the selection of specifically language-impaired subjects. *Journal of Speech & Hearing Disorders, 55*, 468–475.

McCauley, R. J., & Swisher, L. (1984). Use and misuse of norm-referenced tests in clinical assessment: A hypothetical case. *Journal of Speech & Hearing Disorders, 49*, 338–348.

McNeil, M. R., Doyle, P. J., Fossett, T. R. D., & Park, G. H. (2001). Reliability and concurrent validity of the information unit scoring metric for the story retelling procedure. *Aphasiology, 15*(10/11), 991–1006.

Miller, J. F. (1996). Progress in assessing, describing, and defining child language disorder. In N. Cole Kevin, S. Dale Philip, & J. Thal Donna (Eds.), *Assessment of communication and language* (Vol. 6, pp. 309–324). Baltimore: Paul H. Brookes.

Muma, J. R. (1998). Clinical assessment: Description. In *Effective speech-language pathology: A cognitive socialization approach.* Mahwah, NJ: Lawrence Erlbaum. (pp. 166–234). Mahwah, NJ: Lawrence Erlbaum Associates.

Nicholas, L. E., & Brookshire, R. H. (1993). A system for quantifying the informativeness and efficiency of the connected speech of adults with aphasia. *Journal of Speech & Hearing Research, 36*, 338–350.

O'Brian, N., O'Brian, S., Packman, A., & Onslow, M. (2003). Generalizability Theory I: Assessing reliability of observational data in the communication sciences. *Journal of Speech, Language, and Hearing Research, 46*(3), 711–717.

Onslow, M., & Ingham, R. J. (1987). Speech quality measurement and the management of stuttering. *Journal of Speech & Hearing Disorders, 52*(1), 2–17.

Penn, C. (1985). The profile of communicative appropriateness: A clinical tool for the assessment of pragmatics. *South African Journal of Communication Disorders, 32*, 18–23.

Prutting, C. A. (1982). Pragmatics as social competence. *Journal of Speech & Hearing Disorders, 47*, 123–134.

Prutting, C. A., & Kirchner, D. M. (1983). Applied pragmatics. In T. M. Gallagher & C. A. Prutting (Eds.), *Pragmatic assessment and intervention issues in language.* San Diego, CA: College-Hill.

Prutting, C. A., & Kirchner, D. M. (1987). A clinical appraisal of the pragmatic aspects of language. *Journal of Speech and Hearing Disorders, 52*(2), 105–119.

Records, N. L., & Tomblin, J. B. (1994). Clinical decision-making: Describing the decision rules of practicing speech-language pathologists. *Journal of Speech & Hearing Research, 37*, 144–156.

Ringel, R. L., Trachtman, L. E., & Prutting, C. A. (1984, December). The science in human communication sciences. *ASHA,* 35–37.

Roulstone, S. (1997). What's driving you? A template which underpins the assessment of preschool children by speech and language therapists. *European Journal of Disorders of Communication, 32*(3), 299–315.

Ruiz, N. T. (1995a). The social construction of ability and disability: I. Profile types of Latino children identified as language learning disabled. *Journal of Learning Disabilities, 28*(8), 476–490.

Ruiz, N. T. (1995b). The social construction of ability and disability: II. Optimal and at-risk lessons in a bilingual special education classroom. *Journal of Learning Disabilities, 28*(8), 491–502.

Shohamy, E. (1998). Critical language testing and beyond. *Studies in Educational Evaluation, 24*(4), 331–345.

Shohamy, E. (2001a). Democratic assessment as an alternative. *Language Testing, 18*(4), 373–391.

Shohamy, E. (2001b). *The power of tests: A critical perspective on the uses of language tests.* Harlow, UK: Pearson Education.

Shohamy, E. (2004). Reflections on research guidelines, categories, and responsibility. *TESOL Quarterly, 38*(4), 728–731.

Siegel, G. M. (1987). The limits of science in communication disorders. *Journal of Speech & Hearing Disorders, 52,* 306–311.

Siegel, G. M., & Ingham, R. J. (1987). Theory and science in communication disorders. *Journal of Speech & Hearing Disorders, 52,* 99–104.

Simmons-Mackie, N., & Damico, J. S. (2001). Intervention outcomes: A clinical application of qualitative methods. *Topics in Language Disorders, 21*(4), 21–36.

Simmons-Mackie, N., Threats, T. T., & Kagan, A. (2005). Outcome assessment in aphasia: A survey. *Journal of Communication Disorders, 38,* 1–27.

Smith, J. (2005). *Jacques Derrida: Live theory.* New York: Continuum.

Thompson, C. K. (2006). Single subject controlled experiments in aphasia: The science and the state of the science. *Journal of Communication Disorders, 39,* 266–291.

Thomson, J. (2003). Clinical discourse analysis: One theory or many? *Advances in Speech-Language Pathology, 5,* 41–49.

Thomson, J. (2005). Theme analysis of narratives produced by children with and without specific language impairment. *Clinical Linguistics & Phonetics, 19*(3), 175–190.

Usher, R. (2000). Deconstructive happening, ethical moment. In H. Simons & R. Usher (Eds.), *Situated ethics in educational research* (pp. 162–185). London: Routledge-Falmer.

Vanhalle, C., Lemieux, S., Joubert, S., Goulet, P., Ska, B., & Joanette, Y. (2000). Processing of speech acts by right hemisphere brain-damaged patients: An ecological approach. *Aphasiology, 14*(11), 1127–1142.

Wall, D. (1997). Impact and washback in language testing. In C. Clapham & D. Corson (Eds.), *Encyclopedia of language and education: Language testing and assessment* (Vol. 7, pp. 291–302). Dordrecht: Kluwer.

Wolfram Cox, J. (1999). *Triangulation in postpositivist research: A review.* Melbourne, Victoria, Australia Department of Management Working Paper 19/99, Faculty of Business & Economics, Monash University.

Worrall, L. (1999). *Functional communication therapy planner.* Oxon, UK: Winslow Press.

Worrall, L. (2000). The influence of professional values on the functional communication approach in aphasia. In L. Worrall & C. Frattali (Eds.), *Neurogenic communication disorders: A functional approach* (pp. 191–205). New York: Thieme.

Worrall, L. (2006). Professionalism and functional outcomes. *Journal of Communication Disorders, 39,* 320–327.

Worrall, L., Davidson, B., Hersh, D., Howe, T., Ferguson, A., & Sherratt, S. (2006). *What people with aphasia want: Toward person-centred goal-setting in aphasia rehabilitation.* Research in progress. Unpublished manuscript.

Worrall, L., & Egan, J. (2001). A survey of outcome measures used by Australian speech pathologists. *Asia Pacific Journal of Speech, Language and Hearing, 6,* 149–162.

Worrall, L., McCooey, R., Davidson, B., Larkins, B., & Hickson, L. (2002). The validity of functional assessments of communication and the Activity/Participation components of the ICIDH-2: Do they reflect what really happens in real-life? *Journal of Communication Disorders, 35,* 107–137.

3

The Process of Assessment: Discourse Is Dynamic

The current literature in speech-language pathology emphasizes the need for assessment to be both ongoing and integrated within other types of contact with the child or adult with a communication disorder, but the complexities involved in these clinical processes at the expert level have remained largely unexamined. As discussed in Chapter 2, the clinical reasoning process involves a process of triangulation in which the interpretations derived from multiple sources of empirical data are compared and contrasted. The clinician is involved in a "for practical purposes" process of situated problem-solving in weighing the significance of each interpretation to the task at hand, whether that is to determine the presence or nature of a disorder or difficulty or to formulate a therapy plan. As also discussed in Chapter 2, just as it is rare for this process of triangulation to be described in relevant documents, it also is rare for the clinical reasoning processes involved in considering multiple sources of information to be discussed explicitly.

Certain clinical situations typically are seen as challenging and often are regarded as potentially benefiting from consultation with expert speech-language pathologists. Three representative clinical scenarios are discussed in this chapter: assessment for medico-legal purposes, so-called higher-level language assessment, and assessment of bilingual speakers. One reason sometimes offered for the perceived difficulty in such instances is the requirement for skills or information not typically encountered in everyday practice, but more careful consideration suggests otherwise: Although legal situations may be unfamiliar to the speech-language pathologist, for example, the demands of the assessment are limited to everyday skills and professional judgment; higher-level language assessment involves assessment of language well within the scope and level of the practitioner; and although the speech-language pathologist may not know another language, multilingual caseloads are common in current practice. So what is it that sign-posts these clinical situations as challenging? It is suggested that each of these situations forces the speech-language pathologist away from reliance on standardized assessment, because such assessments either are not available or are clearly inappropriate, necessarily pushing the focus toward informal assessment processes, with all of their uncertainty and need for individualized decision-making. In particular, the informal assessment process involved in each of these situations requires grappling with discourse-level assessment of the client. Furthermore, each of these situations requires the recognition that discourse is *dynamic*—that is, shifting and changing. Finally, each of these situations involves the clinician in professional discourses beyond that of speech-language pathology.

For each of the main topics addressed, a critical perspective is offered to allow for further consideration of the issues involved.

Assessment for Medicolegal Purposes

When the term *medicolegal* is mentioned in the context of clinical practice, most speech-language pathologists probably think of a one-time written assessment requested by a legal practitioner handling a compensation claim before the courts for a person with a communication or swallowing disability resulting from some acquired injury. The role of *expert witness* possibly is the next most frequently recognized medicolegal situation in which speech-language pathologists may become involved, such as in presenting an opinion to the court regarding an assessment in a case with which the professional may have been involved as a therapist, or about which the professional is being asked to comment (based on available medical

records) (Critchley, 1970; Silverman, 1992). Although the available research in this area is very limited, some guidelines have emerged regarding the role of the speech-language pathologist as an expert witness in cases involving determination of testamentary capacity (Enderby, 1994; Ferguson et al., 2003; Udell, Sullivan, & Schlanger, 1980). This role tends not to be commonly encountered for most speech-language pathologists, and some private practitioners tend to specialize more in this kind of work. Some preliminary research (Duffield, Ferguson, & Worrall, 2007; Ferguson et al., 2004; Ferguson, Worrall, & McPhee, 2005), however, suggests that speech-language pathologists—certainly those working with persons with acquired neurological disorders—are involved in more frequent and more varied roles in assessments involving medicolegal issues than just testamentary capacity. In this ongoing research, ten speech-language pathologists were interviewed about one or more incidents related to legal decision-making that they had experienced when working with a person with aphasia. The main incidents that were reported included those related to financial decisions, power of attorney, and guardianship. In all but one of the incidents recounted, the issues centered on a situation of conflict between the person with aphasia and family members or friends, or the multidisciplinary team. In the types of situations described, the speech-language pathologist typically was present as a communication facilitator in discussions between a person with aphasia and a legal practitioner, as a consultant for the rehabilitation team seeking to ascertain the wishes of a person with global aphasia, and as an advocate for the rights of people with aphasia to remain independent in decision-making.

The following discussion on this topic looks first at the multiple sources of information to be integrated and what is known about this process; second, at the discourse of the client and how it is assessed; and third, at the wider scope of discourse in which the speech-language pathologist becomes involved.

Integration of Multiple Sources of Information

The types of information that are drawn on in assessment for medicolegal purposes include case history (medical and social) information collected either *directly* from the person with the disorder or an informant (such as a caregiver) or *indirectly* from medical records and the written reports of other professionals and also direct observations made through formal or informal (or both) assessment processes. The guidelines offered by Critchley (1970) and Enderby (1994) clearly stress the importance of using informal observation methods, rather than relying solely on standardized assessment. In fact, as suggested by one group of investigators, informal observations of functional language use may hold greater weight as "evidence" in the legal system (Ferguson et al., 2003). Their study included a case in which a woman had changed her will after the onset of severe aphasia. After her death, one of her adult children challenged this will on the grounds of questionable testamentary capacity. The will was upheld, but one of the points of interest for

speech-language pathologists was the judge's explicit accounting of how he had weighed the different sources of information. He attached great importance to reports by witnesses of communicative interactions that they had with the woman, from which he gauged that with assistance she would be able to convey her wishes and to check that these had been carried out. The judge explicitly discounted the arguments put forward by the expert witness (neuropsychologist) based on test result data abstracted from the medical record.

When speech-language pathologists are assessing an adult (or a child) in any situation, including those concerning medicolegal issues, how do they weigh and integrate multiple sources of information? As seen in Chapter 2, a gap may exist between idealized and actual practice in this regard: Idealized practice suggests that the process is forward and linear, in that it involves collection of preliminary data from a case history; formulation of a hypothesis or set of hypotheses regarding the presence, nature, or severity or impact of the disorder; systematic collection of data designed to allow support or refutation of these hypotheses; and consideration and interpretation of the findings in relation to the hypotheses to form a conclusion. Actual practice may be more end-goal–focused, and therefore "backward" and nonlinear, in that it may involve a determination of the purpose of the assessment (in relation to the referral), selection of what might be described as high-yield assessment strategies (that is, ones that enable observation of multiple aspects in the shortest possible time) designed to provide information needed to attain the end-goal, and consideration and interpretation of findings in relation to the end-goal. The idealized *linear* approach represents assessment as a product achieved after a sequence of steps, whereas in the proposed actual *nonlinear* approach, assessment is recognized as a dynamic process, involving reiterative and ongoing phases, which are essentially open-ended, ceasing only in relation to client or institutional determinations of "goal achieved."

Assessment of the Client's Discourse

In considering the end-goal of an assessment that involves medicolegal issues, the speech-language pathologist inevitably is led to look at dynamic aspects of discourse. Questions about communication in relation to testamentary capacity, for example, concern whether and how the person could have communicated appropriate instructions and whether that person could have checked that the will accurately represented those instructions before signing it. To address such questions, information is needed about how much the person understands personally relevant information in context and whether the person recognizes that he or she is not comprehending information, and how the person goes about requesting clarification or confirmation of information. Information is needed about how much the person can convey about what sorts of things, and whether the person knows when the intended message has been "delivered," and how the person goes about repairing communication breakdowns. For example, what does the person do when he or she cannot find the word—does the person use gesture or drawing, and does this assist? And what can a communication partner do to assist? In a situation in which a speech-language pathologist knows that a person with aphasia is making a will and wants to ensure that the records of assessment be as comprehensive as possible in case of some potential challenge to testamentary capacity, use of a combination of the following information is recommended (Ferguson et al., 2003): results from the full administration of the Western Aphasia Battery (Kertesz, 2006), along with transcribed representative discourse samples of interaction, and clear statements regarding the communication strategies required by partners to facilitate effective communication.

In situations in which the speech-language pathologist is conducting an assessment for compensation purposes, then the questions are not only about how the person's communication has been impaired but also about the impact of the communication disability on everyday living and the nature of the supports likely to be needed. So, for example, how will the person communicate in the workplace or in an academic setting—how does the person manage negotiation or clarification? In situations of the sort revealed in the study (mentioned previously) which involved interviewing 10 speech-language pathologists about critical incidents in relation to legal matters in their practice (Duffield, Ferguson, & Worrall, 2007; Ferguson et al., 2004; Ferguson, Worrall, & McPhee, 2005), the speech-language pathologists recounted how they were involved in moment-to-moment assessment as they acted as facilitators of communication between the person with the communication disability and others. In both types of situations, it appears that direct observation of interactive discourse within natural contexts is best suited to the demands of assessment for medicolegal purposes.

Beyond the Discourse of Speech-Language Pathology

In the discourse of speech-language pathology, the term *evidence* is used within the scientific paradigm to encapsulate observations that can be demonstrated and tested empirically. In the legal paradigm, however, *evidence* refers to the accounts offered by persons of what they witnessed or the contextually relevant artifacts of events (such as a weapon at the scene of a crime). In other words, *evidence* within the legal system is far closer to the qualitative postpositivist interpretive paradigm, in which accounts are recognized as interpretations. In the legal system, the judge or jury weighs (triangulates) the multiple interpretations to arrive at a determination of what appears to be a convergent interpretation or judgment. Although an expert witness may be asked by the court to provide information or to express an opinion (depending on the legal system of the country), this information or opinion becomes one of the sources of evidence to be taken into account in the judgment of others. This is not to suggest that a scientific basis for expert evidence is not required, because in recent years, in many countries the scientific paradigm increasingly has become an important consideration in the extent to which tests conducted by

expert witnesses are considered to be reliable (Olsson, 2004a; Stygall, 2001), but rather to emphasize that expert evidence is itself one more account for the court's consideration.

The legal system has been a venue for considerable linguistic inquiry (Gibbons, 2003a; Olsson, 2004b) because it is a system in which sociocultural power is enacted through language (Bourdieu, 1991; Fairclough, 1989). The most obvious criticisms in relation to language and the law relate to the complexity and specificity of language use that render much of its meanings opaque to the layperson. Of greater significance, a critical linguistic perspective has highlighted the complex issues relating to the balance of power during interactions in police interviews (Haworth, 2006), and during the highly structured genre of courtroom examination (Chang, 2004; Eades, 2000), and persisting in less structured legal dispute resolution procedures (Candlin & Maley, 1994). An analysis of expert testimony from a critical discourse perspective has suggested an ongoing power struggle between science and the law, observable through the unique discourse practices afforded to expert witnesses (longer turns, the use of hedges without loss of credibility, and the use of discourse markers of contrast and conclusion) (Stygall, 2001). The inequities associated with language use in legal interactions are magnified for people with difficulties with speech who use alternative and augmentative communication systems (Huer & Yaniv, 2006) and for persons with difficulties with language (including children, people who speak a different language, and the hearing-impaired) (Gibbons, 2003b).

Higher-Level Language Assessment

Assessments tapping into what is referred to as higher-level or high-level language are typically unpublished informal protocols, such as the Mt. Wilga Test for Higher Level Language Function (Christie, Clarke, & Mortensen, 1986). Such assessment protocols generally involve the client in inferential comprehension of lengthy and detailed passages read aloud, following long and syntactically complex instructions; verbal and written descriptions or explanations; metalinguistic reflections on grammaticality and meanings of words and proverbs or idioms; meta-pragmatic reflections on appropriateness of hypothetical social scenarios; and problem-solving involving verbal reasoning, sometimes including calculation. The term *higher-level* or *high-level* generally refers to uses of language that are seen as complex in some way that relates to aspects of cognition (attention, perception, memory, convergent-divergent thinking, executive function), but these aspects of cognition typically are ill defined. Other language assessments, that is, those that are not described as "higher level," usually attempt to incorporate tasks that are able to be completed with ease by most people within the range of normal intelligence (as measured by intelligence quotient [IQ]) in the population, and on which performance is relatively unaffected by level of education. Higher-level language assessments assume a "world knowledge" associated with particular social demographics. For example, particular assessment items such as idioms or proverbs may be more or less recognizable to different age cohorts as a result of the socio-cultural shifts occurring over different generations. Higher-level language tasks usually are affected by cognitive ability and education level and experience (for example, familiarity with purposes of testing and identifying the type of answer sought). These sociocultural influences mean that higher-level assessment is influenced by socioeconomic demographics (social class), with a strong bias to middle class content and expectations. The reference standard for such assessments usually is taken to be an estimate of the previous level of functioning of the person (in the case of acquired brain damage), or an estimate of how another person in a similar age cohort and social demographic would perform on the assessment (assessment of unaffected siblings is a strongly recommended procedure to provide such an estimate).

As in the preceding section, the following discussion of this topic looks first at the multiple sources of information to be integrated and what is known about how this process is done; second, at the discourse of the client and how it is assessed, and third, at the wider scope of discourse in which the speech-language pathologist becomes involved.

Integration of Multiple Sources of Information

In considering the range of information that can fall within the scope of a higher-level language assessment (as described previously), the question arises as to how such disparate information is integrated for the purposes of the assessment. After conducting such protocols of observation and sampling, the speech-language pathologist is faced with many pieces of information about what the client can or cannot do. The close links between higher-level language use and cognitive processing also prompt the speech-language pathologist to consider how the client goes about each task—for example, is processing slow or perhaps inefficient. with multiple attempts before a final response, or does the client impulsively respond or show latency of response? The idealized conception of how this information is integrated is that each of these observations is to be seen as a reflection of a general model of cognition and cognitive processing that is hierarchical in nature, such that problems with lower-level cognitive functions such as attention, perception, and memory will affect higher-level cognition, and hence language. Thus, in the case of traumatic brain injury, the "highest" level of language problems (those involving verbal reasoning for executive functions such as social judgment) may arise from very fundamental problems (such as not remembering the information on which judgment is needed), or from problems arising at that same level of cognition (such as inability to weigh consequences, for example). In the case of aphasia from stroke, the "highest" level of language problem observed (incoherence in verbal reasoning) typically would arise from problems with convergent and divergent naming processes. The speech-language pathologist faces a dilemma in formulating intervention for higher-level language problems: whether to work at the level of the deficit (for example, memory and semantic retrieval),

looking for effects on verbal reasoning performance, or whether to work directly on verbal reasoning, finding ways to facilitate or compensate for the lower-level difficulty. In actual practice, the speech-language pathologist faces an even greater challenge in that it is not feasible to assess every possible aspect of cognition to yield more than an informed estimate of function, so the clinician must assess selectively. This selective assessment may be shaped by the end-goals of high-level clients more prominently than in other situations, in light of the clients' power in the clinical interaction as a result of being able to use language with sufficient proficiency to negotiate. Based on a selective assessment, the clinician's directions for intervention are shaped by these constrained findings and the client's goals, and further research could illuminate these processes.

Assessment of the Client's Discourse

Two points that are particularly relevant to the assessment of the client's discourse at the higher levels of language are (1) what constitutes the natural use of higher-level language and (2) how dynamic aspects of higher level language may be ascertained.

In the protocols generally used to assess higher level language, the tasks often seem rarified and to lack face validity, with both clients and clinicians often excusing difficulties on the basis that the task is unusual or not typically experienced by the client. This attitude presumes that higher-level language is not involved in everyday situations, however, and also may reflect educated middle class assumptions about the complexity of language use demanded in interactions between less educated people from lower-level socioeconomic groups. For example, workers on a building site need to negotiate continually in order to manage multiple tasks across multiple persons with various degrees of experience and backgrounds, communicating against competing noise and activity with high time pressures. Humor with its demands for inference and acutely judged timing and contextual requirements arises universally. It is possible for a person to struggle with a metalinguistic interpretation of proverb or idiom while recognizing double meanings conveyed in television advertising and exploiting these for their joke potential. Of interest, when the list of the observed everyday activities observed in the natural lives of people with aphasia is considered (Davidson, Worrall, & Hickson, 2003; Worrall, McCooey, Davidson, Larkins, & Hickson, 2002), many of these activities stand out as offering opportunities and demands for higher-level language function—for example, understanding apologies, discussing medical conditions and prior hospital admissions, telling jokes, questioning, managing forms related to medical insurance, and so on. These observations prompt the question as to whether higher-level language is in fact "high" at all, or whether the sensitivity of higher-level language testing to educational level reflects experience with decontextualized assessment tasks, rather than linguistic complexity as such. If everyday language use involves complexity and cognitive demands, then this recognition highlights the need to consider the necessity for the development of theoretical models of cognition that relate to language use in everyday situations.

Missing from the available protocols for higher-level language assessment, however, are methods to sample and analyze interactive discourse—yet interactive discourse is the most commonly encountered challenge faced by people with higher-level language impairment. Although discourse may be elicited interactively in the available protocols, the importance of the dynamic aspects of the discourse is not explored, despite the fact that these aspects allow for shades of meaning to be negotiated (essential for maintaining social harmony in relationships), and for the use of language to recalibrate the power relationship between the person with the language impairment and the communication partner (through, for example, turn-holding and allocation strategies). Published protocols to guide sampling and analysis of conversation are available (Whitworth, Perkins, & Lesser, 1997), and a considerable research base has accrued to suggest the usefulness of diverse methodologies for sampling and analyzing interaction (Armstrong, Ferguson, Mortensen, & Togher, 2005; Cherney, Shadden, & Coelho, 1998; Coelho, Youse, & Le, 2002; Ferguson, 1994, 2000; Milroy & Perkins, 1992; Mortensen, 2005; Prins & Bastiaanse, 2004; Togher, 2001; Togher, Hand, & Code, 1997). These methodologies, however, are not widely used. For example, in a study of outcome measures used in aphasia, only 13 of 336 (3.8%) reported tools involved discourse analysis (Simmons-Mackie, Threats, & Kagan, 2005). This underuse of a relevant assessment methodology by speech-language pathologists may arise from the need to cross into the discourse of formal linguistics—relatively uncomfortable territory for many in the field.

Beyond the Discourse of Speech-Language Pathology

Discourse analysis requires that the speech-language pathologist be able to confidently describe language within paradigms and frameworks derived from theories and approaches from a very different field. Speech-language pathologists are familiar with descriptive approaches to the study of language (Crystal, 1992, 2004; Greenbaum & Quirk, 1990). Professional preparation programs introduce speech-language pathologists to the field of linguistics, so most speech-language pathologists are acquainted with general theories of linguistics, most notably, Chomsky's generative grammar (Cook, 1996), but they typically have little awareness of major competing theories in linguistics, such as lexical-functional grammar (Bresnan, 2001). Likewise, most will have a general concept of sociolinguistics as an area but little awareness of specific theories or approaches within that field. Thus, speech-language pathologists often understand and use linguistic terminology in ways that do not reflect their theoretical origins (for example, the use of the term *pragmatics* to imply a level of language, rather than a theoretical perspective) and apply linguistic theories in ways that distort fundamental constructs (for example, the use of Grice's maxims as normative prescriptions). Thus, the "discourse about discourse" in the field of speech-language pathology often is both confused and confusing to practitioners, other professionals, and clients. On the other hand, the field of speech-language pathology has taken on board much that is useful from the field of linguistics in its applications to language testing and monologic discourse analyses. Unfortunately, the illuminations offered by linguistic approaches to the analysis of dynamic aspects of discourse remain underutilized.

At a more concrete level, lack of time is the reason most often given for why speech-language pathologists do not undertake discourse analysis (particularly of natural interactions involving a partner other than a clinician, or involving monologic discourse longer than 1- to 2-minute samples). Obtaining natural samples, however, is as easy as sending a small audio recorder home with a client, and the transcription process is itself a vital part of the analytical-interpretive process (Ochs, 1979; Psathas & Anderson, 1990) that provides much information to the clinician, even before any further linguistic analysis. The availability of relatively inexpensive and easy-to-use computerized software to conduct automated basic interactive analyses allows for basic analyses within minutes (Miller, 1996, 2003). Further linguistic coding and analysis do depend on the individual clinician's knowledge of particular linguistic frameworks, but with a selective end-goal focus, such analysis can be conducted within a reasonable time frame. Also, discourse analysis, particularly for the dynamic aspects, does not necessarily need to be based on transcription. Transcription transforms the discourse from a time-bound flow to a static product, so in many ways it provides a distorted view of what is going on. For example, the reader of a transcript can look ahead to see what the outcome of repair will be, but the person in an unfolding interaction knows only what has gone before and works within that understanding. Online observation of selected dynamic aspects of the interaction (e.g., appeals for assistance versus other repair versus self-repair) in real-world situations (e.g., workplace, home, or school visit) may provide more opportunities to sample and analyze authentic language use.

Certainly, the processes just described for the assessment of dynamic aspects of discourse do not require any more time for assessment than that required in the administration, scoring, analysis, and interpretation of standardized assessment methods. Why, then, the lack of uptake? Possibly, this situation could reflect a power struggle between discourses of data. Paradoxically, the closer the observation is to the actual experience, the less it is valued as "data." So observing a partner supply the word for the person with the communication problem is an observation but not data, whereas clinician-applied prompts for word-finding difficulty in a test *are* data. A requirement in the discourse of data is that a piece of data be an abstraction, a transformed moment —transformed from the actual event to the recordable event. Data thus constitute a symbol, an index, that stands in place of the actual phenomenon: The more abstract, the more symbolic; the less representational, the more "data-like." The abstract nature of data confers inherent symbolic power—data

can take on meanings over and above whatever the data may represent. So data from standardized tests, for example, become transformed into means and standard deviations and percentiles, which come to represent "normal" and "abnormal." Data from discourse analysis also are derived from a transformation (for example, from interaction to transcription); therefore, as previously mentioned, transcriptions also need to be regarded as indexical and interpretive.

Bilingual/Multilingual[1] Assessment

In this chapter, the issues related to bilingual assessment allow a look at two further aspects of the dynamic nature of discourse, explored later in this book: Discourse changes (1) with contexts of situation and (2) over time (see also Chapters 5 and 8 for further discussion of bilingual issues). Naturally, such dynamic changes occur for any speaker, but these changes are especially significant in assessment of bilingual speakers.

Following the pattern of previous sections, this section looks first, at the multiple sources of information to be integrated and what is known about how this process is accomplished; second, at the discourse of the client and how it is assessed; and third, at the wider scope of discourse in which the speech-language pathologist becomes involved.

---

[1]From this point on the term *bilingual* is used to include "multilingual" speakers and does not exclude this population.

Integration of Multiple Sources of Information

As with any assessment, the speech-language pathologist assessing a bilingual speaker will be integrating multiple sources of information including case history, formal and informal assessments, and reports from client, family, teachers, and so on. The contextual variation known to occur for bilingual speakers becomes a specific aspect of the assessment, however, because the speaker can be expected to use different languages for different purposes in different situations (i.e., field) and with different partners (i.e., tenor) and may use different languages in different ways (i.e., mode)—for example, in shifting languages within formal and less formal registers. Speakers also may make use of the resource of code-shifting, so that they can switch from one language to another in order to capture a particular shade of meaning or expression unavailable in the other language (either unavailable to the speaker or unavailable in the linguistic system of that language) (Lanza, 2004; Piller, 2002). Speech-language pathologists assessing bilingual children can expect ongoing changes in patterns and specific features of both languages, so they need to tailor their assessment to capture such changes of significance. Some of these changes will be developmental, just as with monolingual children, and some of the changes may be associated with attrition (as in the case of a first language if unused) or associated with learning as the child or adult develops increased proficiency in a second language. Speech-language pathologists involved in the assessment of bilingual adults with acquired language impairment also anticipate that their assessment will need to capture expected changes associated with recovery.

Having obtained information from multiple sources that allow for identification of changes with contexts of situation and over time, the speech-language pathologist faces questions in comparing the information from one language to other, to decide whether either or both languages show problems. Comparisons with monolingual speakers have been challenged as invalid in the literature on children because considerable evidence suggests that language development and learning in bilingual speakers occur in ways that are significantly different from those for monolingual speakers (Stow & Dodd, 2003). Obtaining normative reference groups for bilingual children is complex and, arguably, beside the point. Comparison across contexts generates considerable information for the clinician to use in determining maximum language performance and in identifying when language use is compromised. Thus, such comparisons allow for "dynamic assessment" (Merritt, 1998; Pena, Iglesias, & Lidz, 2001), with the term *dynamic* used here in the sense of a repeated assessment that shows potential for learning and possible ways in which performance may be facilitated.

This challenge also holds for adult speakers, with most speech-language pathologists adopting the comparison point as the estimated premorbid pattern of language use, making use of patient and family reports to assist in this estimation. Estimating attrition (the extent to which the person's proficiency with the first language has been eroded over time) becomes another part of this guesswork (Seliger & Vago,

1991). The substantial literature on differential recovery of languages for bilingual speakers informs the considerations for assessment of languages over time (Paradis, 2004), whereas the assessment across contexts for adult speakers often is used to inform very critical decisions regarding the language in which therapy will be provided (Roberts, 2001).

Assessment of the Client's Discourse

In both adults and children, the speech-language pathologist's assessment needs to be designed to capture changes across contexts and over time, and this demands replicable assessment methodologies. Replicability is associated with standardization, so a strong impetus exists to use assessment tools for their standardization despite questions regarding the inadequacies of their translation, cultural inappropriateness of their content, and the inapplicability of their normative reference pool. As previously discussed, discourse assessments can allow for the demands of replication and can provide for culturally appropriate content and individualized analysis and interpretation. Issues regarding adequacy of translation or interpretation of discourse necessarily remain an issue for discourse assessment. Also, caution is needed because types of discourse are highly contextualized within the culture of their use: For example, the narrative structures described in much of the speech-language pathology literature are associated with Western culture and differ from those associated with other cultures (Bamberg, 1997). As with all aspects of working with people from other cultures, the speech-language pathologist needs a constant awareness of the potential for difference and a critical stance in order to identify culturally based assumptions and concepts.

Some evidence emerging in the research literature points to inequities in access to speech-language pathology services for bilingual speakers (Stow & Dodd, 2003). In particular, the research suggests that the process of assessment in bilingual speakers is less than ideal in both languages, and after assessment, these clients may be less likely to receive adequate intervention (Winter, 1999). For example, Kritikos (2003) conducted a U.S. survey with 811 participating speech-language pathologists from five states. An important result from the survey was that 40% reported that they would be less likely to refer a child "with bilingual input" for intervention than a child "who hears only one language" (p. 85). Kritikos argues: "Clearly, the most accurate, comprehensive, and culturally appropriate language assessment is useless if the interpretation and decision-making phase of the process is biased. . . . If bilingual individuals are less likely to be recommended for or provided services, even by SLPs with more diverse backgrounds, this is a significant problem for the profession" (Kritikos, 2003, pp. 85–86).

Beyond the Discourse of Speech-Language Pathology

Assessment of bilingual speakers moves speech-language pathologists into the different discourses associated with different cultures, not simply the different linguistic codes used within the discourse. Speech-language pathologists with greater knowledge of both other cultures and other languages appear to be more confident to take on the challenges involved in bilingual assessment. For example, Kritikos (2003) found that speech-language pathologists who had experience of learning a second language as part of their cultural experience (real-world learning) reported greater belief in their personal efficacy compared with those who had learned a second language within the context of an academic program, and this latter group reported greater belief in their personal efficacy compared with monolingual speech-language pathologists.

Dynamic Assessment: Implications for Practice

One of the problems with a relativist position with regard to assessment, such as that presented throughout this chapter, is that speech-language pathologists are left to ask, "Well, then, does this person have a problem?" For example, is it sufficient that the client or the caregiver identifies the client as having a communication disorder? As discussed in Chapter 2, a midway point in this kind of debate is offered through the suggestion from the literature on expertise in context (Agnew, Ford, & Hayes, 1997), in that the benefits of scientific thinking can be harnessed to examine critically the assessment evidence toward an interpretation for practical purpose. So, rather than just asking "Is there evidence to support that this person has a communication disorder?" (positive), speech-language pathologists also should attempt to actively look for evidence to falsify the

hypothesis: "Is there evidence that does not support the presence of disorder?" (negative). It also should be possible to build into the assessment process ways to consider false positives or false negatives—for example, through review of not only positive identifications but also of negative identifications. This same thinking applies not just to presence-absence decisions but also to attempts to describe the nature of particular problems and their effects on the life of the person. Obviously, it is important to look for evidence suggesting specific communication or swallowing disorders and to characterize the relative severity of such problems if detected. But it is equally important to look for evidence that would counter such conclusions, and to conduct appropriate follow-up to check for faulty description. This type of process allows a systematic way to integrate the information derived from multiple sources, so that rather than comparing source with source (seeking some kind of answer to which one is "more right"), the comparative process is about which parts of the information provided (from whatever source) inform this scientific decision making process. In medicolegal assessment, such a process would provide the kind of "evidence" that would inform the judgments required from the legal system, and required in advocacy for people with communication disorders who have been or are at risk of being at a disadvantage in that system. In higher-level language assessment, such a process would allow greater confidence in making individualized judgments in relation to "guestimates" of previous or comparable language function. In bilingual language assessment, such a process would allow greater confidence in making individualized judgments in relation to presence or absence of problems in different languages and the relative significance of such problems.

With respect to the dynamic aspects of discourse and the challenges faced by speech-language pathologists in integrating these within complex assessment processes, a critical perspective has shown points at which people with communication disorders are at particular risk of unfair treatment at both the hands of others (for example, in the legal system) and our own profession (for example, services for bilingual speakers). Also, this perspective has highlighted how cultural biases within the profession shape the content of assessment (for example, class bias in the content of higher-level assessment). The considerations and suggestions in this chapter support the movement in the field toward the recognition of the importance of dynamic assessment and has suggested some ways in which the dynamic aspects of discourse can be captured in such an approach. Fundamental to such a process of assessment is the recognition that the notion of data (and what sorts of data are of value) is a cultural product.

References

Agnew, N. M., Ford, K. M., & Hayes, P. J. (1997). Expertise in context: Personally constructed, socially selected and reality-relevant? In P. J. Feltovich, K. M. Ford, & R. R. Hoffman (Eds.), *Expertise in context: Human and machine* (pp. 220–244). Menlo Park, CA: AAAI Press/MIT Press.

Armstrong, E., Ferguson, A., Mortensen, L., & Togher, L. (2005). Acquired language disorders: Some functional insights. In R. Hasan, J. Webster, & C. Matthiessen (Eds.), *Continuing discourse on language* (Vol. 1). London: Equinox.

Bamberg, M. (Ed.). (1997). *Narrative development: Six approaches.* Mahwah, NJ: Lawrence Erlbaum Associates.

Bourdieu, P. (1991). *Language and symbolic power* (G. Raymond & M. Adamson, Trans.). Oxford: Polity Press.

Bresnan, J. (2001). *Lexical-functional syntax.* Malden, MA: Blackwell.

Candlin, C. N., & Maley, Y. (1994). Framing the dispute. *International Journal for the Semiotics of Law, 7*(19), 75–98.

Chang, Y. (2004). Courtroom questioning as a culturally situated persuasive genre of talk. *Discourse & Society, 15*(6), 705–722.

Cherney, L. R., Shadden, B. B., & Coelho, C. A. (Eds.). (1998). *Analyzing discourse in communicatively impaired adults.* Gaithersburg, MD: Aspen.

Christie, J., Clarke, W., & Mortensen, L. (1986). *Mt. Wilga test for higher level language functioning.* Unpublished manuscript, Mt. Wilga Rehabilitation Centre, Sydney.

Coelho, C., Youse, K. M., & Le, K. N. (2002). Conversational discourse in closed-head-injured and non-brain-injured adults. *Aphasiology, 16*(4/5/6), 659–672.

Cook, V. J. (1996). *Chomsky's universal grammar: An introduction.* Oxford: Blackwell.

Critchley, M. (1970). *Aphasiology* (pp. 288–295). London: Edward Arnold.

Crystal, D. (1992). *Profiling linguistic disability.* London: Whurr.

Crystal, D. (2004). *Rediscover grammar.* Harlow, UK: Pearson Longman.

Davidson, B., Worrall, L., & Hickson, L. (2003). Identifying communication activities of older people with aphasia: Evidence from naturalistic observation. *Aphasiology, 17*(3), 243–264.

Duffield, G., Ferguson, A., & Worrall, L. (2007). *Legal issues and aphasia: Critical incidents for speech pathologists.* Paper presented at the Speech Pathology Australia national conference, Sydney, May 27–31.

Eades, D. (2000). I don't think it's an answer to the question: Silencing Aboriginal witnesses in court. *Language in Society*, 29(2), 161–195.

Enderby, P. (1994). The testamentary capacity of dysphasic patients. *Medico-Legal Journal*, 62(2), 70–80.

Fairclough, N. (1989). *Language and power*. London: Longman.

Ferguson, A. (1994). The influence of aphasia, familiarity and activity on conversational repair. *Aphasiology*, 8(2), 143–157.

Ferguson, A. (2000). Maximising communicative effectiveness. In N. Muller (Ed.), *Pragmatic approaches to aphasia* (pp. 53–88). Amsterdam: John Benjamins.

Ferguson, A., Worrall, L., & McPhee, J. (2005). *Communicating legal issues: Facilitating access to justice for people with aphasia*. Paper presented at the 3rd International Conference on Communication, Medicine & Ethics, Sydney, June 30–Jul. 2.

Ferguson, A., Worrall, L., McPhee, J., Buskell, R., Armstrong, E., & Togher, L. (2003). Testamentary capacity and aphasia: A descriptive case report with implications for clinical practice. *Aphasiology*, 17(10), 965–980.

Ferguson, A., Worrall, L., McPhee, J., Buskell, R., Armstrong, E., & Togher, L. (2004). *Autonomy in life decisions for people with aphasia: Issues for speech pathologists*. Paper presented at the 26th World Congress of the International Association of Logopedics & Phoniatrics, Brisbane, Australia, 29 Aug. 29–Sept. 2.

Gibbons, J. (2003a). *Forensic linguistics: An introduction to language in the justice system*. Malden, MA: Blackwell.

Gibbons, J. (2003b). Language and disadvantage before the law. In *Forensic linguistics: An introduction to language in the justice system* (pp. 200–227). Malden, MA: Blackwell.

Greenbaum, S., & Quirk, R. (1990). *A student's grammar of the English language*. Harlow, UK: Longman

Haworth, K. (2006). The dynamics of power and resistance in police interview discourse. *Discourse & Society*, 17(6), 739–759.

Huer, M. B., & Yaniv, K. (2006, December). Access to justice: An SLP's guide to helping persons with complex communication needs voice their case. *ASHA Leader*, 6–7, 28–29.

Kertesz, A. (2006). *Western aphasia battery— revised*. San Antonio, TX: Harcourt Assessment.

Kritikos, E. P. (2003). Speech-language pathologists' beliefs about language assessment of bilingual/bicultural individuals. *American Journal of Speech-Language Pathology*, 12(1), 73–91.

Lanza, E. (2004). *Language mixing in infant bilingualism: A sociolinguistic perspective*. Oxford: Oxford University Press.

Merritt, D. (1998). *Language intervention in the classroom*. San Diego, CA: Singular.

Miller, J. F. (1996). Progress in assessing, describing, and defining child language disorder. In K. N. Cole, P. S. Dale, & D. J. Thal (Eds.), *Assessment of communication and language* (Vol. 6, pp. 309–324). Baltimore: Paul H. Brookes.

Miller, J. F. (2003). *Systematic analysis of language transcripts—SALT* (Version V8.0). Madison, WI: Language Analysis Laboratory, University of Wisconsin–Madison.

Milroy, L., & Perkins, L. (1992). Repair strategies in aphasic discourse: Towards a collaborative model. *Clinical Linguistics & Phonetics*, 6, 27–40.

Mortensen, L. (2005). Written discourse and acquired brain impairment: Evaluation of structural and semantic features of personal letters from a Systemic Functional Linguistic perspective. *Clinical Linguistics & Phonetics*, 19(3), 227–247.

Ochs, E. (1979). Transcription as theory. In E. Ochs & B. B. E. Schieffelin (Eds.), *Developmental pragmatics*. New York: Academic Press.

Olsson, J. (2004a). Evidence in court. In *Forensic linguistics: An introduction to language, crime and the law* (pp. 41–48). London: Continuum.

Olsson, J. (2004b). *Forensic linguistics: An introduction to language, crime and the law.* London: Continuum.

Paradis, M. (2004). *A neurolinguistic theory of bilingualism.* Amsterdam: John Benjamins.

Pena, E., Iglesias, A., & Lidz, C. S. (2001). Reducing test bias through dynamic assessment of children's word learning ability. *American Journal of Speech-Language Pathology, 10*(2), 138–154.

Piller, I. (2002). *Bilingual couples talk: The discursive construction of hybridity.* Amsterdam: John Benjamins.

Prins, R., & Bastiaanse, R. (2004). Analysing the spontaneous speech of aphasic speakers. *Aphasiology, 18*(12), 1075–1091.

Psathas, G., & Anderson, T. (1990). The "practices" of transcription in conversation analysis. *Semiotica, 78*(1–2), 75–99.

Roberts, P. M. (2001). Assessment and treatment for bilingual and culturally diverse patients. In R. Chapey (Ed.), *Language intervention strategies in aphasia and related neurogenic communication disorders* (pp. 208–232). Baltimore: Lippincott Williams & Wilkins.

Seliger, H. W., & Vago, R. M. (Eds.). (1991). *First language attrition.* Cambridge: Cambridge University Press.

Silverman, F. H. (1992). *Legal-ethical considerations, restrictions, and obligations for clinicians who treat communicative disorders* (2nd ed.). Springfield, IL: Charles C. Thomas.

Simmons-Mackie, N., Threats, T. T., & Kagan, A. (2005). Outcome assessment in aphasia: A survey. *Journal of Communication Disorders, 38*, 1–27.

Stow, C., & Dodd, B. (2003). Providing an equitable service to bilingual children in the UK: A review. *International Journal of Language & Communication Disorders, 38*(4), 351–377.

Stygall, G. (2001). A different class of witnesses: Experts in the courtroom. *Discourse Studies, 3*(3), 327–349.

Togher, L. (2001). Discourse sampling in the 21st century. *Journal of Communication Disorders, 34*, 131–150.

Togher, L., Hand, L., & Code, C. (1997). Measuring service encounters in the traumatic brain injury population. *Aphasiology, 11*, 491–504.

Udell, R., Sullivan, R. A., & Schlanger, P. H. (1980). Legal competency of aphasic patients: Role of speech-language pathologists. *Archives of Physical Medicine and Rehabilitation, 61*, 374–375.

Whitworth, A., Perkins, L., & Lesser, R. (1997). *Conversation analysis profile for people with aphasia (CAPPA).* London: Whurr.

Winter, K. (1999). Speech and language therapy provision for bilingual children: Aspects of the current service. *International Journal of Language & Communication Disorders, 34*(1), 85–95.

Worrall, L., McCooey, R., Davidson, B., Larkins, B., & Hickson, L. (2002). The validity of functional assessments of communication and the Activity/Participation components of the ICIDH-2: Do they reflect what really happens in real-life? *Journal of Communication Disorders, 35*, 107–137.

4

Service Provision: Discourse and Power

This chapter looks at the relationship between language and power in relation to the provision of speech-language pathology services. The term *power of speech* is a commonly used metaphor in the community to convey the importance of the role of communication in obtaining what people need. This metaphor resonates for all persons involved in speech-language pathology services —clients[1], caregivers, and professionals. The way the discourse of therapeutic interactions displays and creates power relationships between the clinician and the person with a communication disorder is the most transparent opportunity for examining this phenomenon and is the topic of Chapter 6. Here, however, the wider issue of service provision in relation to discourse and power is considered.

Most obviously, speech-language pathologists make decisions about what services are to be provided on the basis of observations about the client's discourse—for example, the nature and severity of difficulties displayed, and the availability of effective interventions for the observed difficulties. Also, the extent to which the client has the opportunity to express his or her needs and desired goals for therapy will shape service provision. Worrall (2000) proposes that speech-language pathologists change the process of decision-making with regard to service provision from a clinician-centered, assessment-first approach (as discussed in Chapter 2) to a client-centered approach. The therapy goals identified by the person with the communication disorder should drive the selection of assessment processes, the therapy process, and the evaluation of the outcome of therapy (Worrall, 2000, 2006; Worrall et al., 2006). In this view, power shifts toward the client from the outset of service provision, and the mechanism for this power shift is through the discourse opportunities provided.

---

[1]This book uses both the terms 'client' and 'patient' to describe the role of persons when participating in services provided by speech-language pathologists and other professionals. The term 'client' has been used generically, but the term 'patient' is used when this role is occurring within a medical environment such as a hospital.

Less obviously, the discourse of clients and their caregivers influences clinicians' perceptions of the competence of the client, and this in turn affects what services are offered. In two case studies, Barton (1999) looks at how an educated parent of a child with attention deficit hyperactivity disorder engages with the clinician, resulting in extended service provision, and compares this outcome with that for a child with cerebral palsy whose parent holds different views from those of the clinician, resulting in a truncated interaction, with provision of little guidance. Barton suggests that clinicians' perceptions of parents' competence to manage their children's problems may arise from the way the parents talk about the problem, particularly in their ability to frame the problem in ways that are compatible with the clinical framework.

Examined in this chapter are how service provision is influenced by discourse and how discourse provides a window into the power relationships involved in service provision. Discussed first is the role of narrative in articulating client perspectives, followed by stories of clinicians exploring how their approaches to service provision have been shaped by such narratives. These perspectives argue for the importance of collaborative or partnership approaches. Also considered in this chapter are issues surrounding empowerment and its relationship to self-help groups and advocacy for services.

Talk as a Way to Redress Power

The difficulties and social consequences of disability are discussed by Goffman (1971, 1990), who makes the point that in general, these difficulties can be redressed by talk, such as through explanation. So-called *invisible disabilities*, however, make redress unavailable; to explain mental health problems, for example, is to alert other persons to the existence of a disorder. Even more complex are invisible disabilities of communication, in which talk to redress the problem instantiates the difficulty—for example, if a person who stutters finds that stuttering is displayed through the explanation. Persons with communication disability find themselves doubly disempowered—first, through the loss of communication itself, and second, through the loss of communication as a means by which the disability can be explained or counteracted. As Mackay (a sociologist with personal experience of aphasia) has noted, "Medical/ablest discrimination of persons with aphasia consists of disapproving of their performance (voice-less-ness) and substituting for performance the word 'incompetence'" (Mackay, 2003, p. 813). The central role of communication in ensuring adequate services and the double disadvantage experienced by persons with communication disability were recognized and integrated in the work of Law and colleagues, who used the experiences of three groups of people affected by communication disability—teenagers with developmental language disorder, adults with communication difficulty associated with learning disability, and adults with aphasia following stroke—to test the adequacy of communication in services offered by general practitioners (Law, Bunning, Byng, Farrelly, & Heyman, 2005). These investigators suggested that if communication is adequate for those with communicative disability, then it is adequate more generally as well.

One of the most important sources of redress for illness and disability is obtained through the telling of the affected person's story or narrative. Frank, perhaps the most well-known writer in this area, sets out the view that the modern, or *positivist*, narrative of illness is one in which medicine solves the problem: a *restitution* narrative (Frank, 1995). In the restitution narrative, the "hero" is the clinician (or the medicine or intervention provided), and the patient is the passive recipient. This story is associated with the medical ideology in which the affected person adopts the role of patient (sick role). The doctor (or medical institution) is an agent of social control, deciding who gets what services. Frank suggests that as medicine and technology have improved, more people are chronically ill or disabled, leading to questions about the relevance of medicine and the centrality of medicine. Chronic illness and long-lasting disability previously have received relatively little attention in medicine, possibly because the tools and strategies of modern medicine had little to offer. Some evidence suggests that this situation is shifting (Lubkin & Larsen, 2006), both in terms of medical recognition and intervention and in terms of recognition of the legitimacy of management outside the medical framework. Frank argues that the postmodern, or *postpositivist*, view captures other voices, other perspectives. He suggests that the *quest* narrative, in which the patient seeks or derives meaning from his or her own experiences, reflects the postmodern view. Thus, many people, although they would prefer not to be facing the challenges of illness or disability, tell of lessons learned or report renewal of a sense of self.

Personal narratives about communication disability are being given increasing prominence in the professional literature but continue to be relatively unusual (Kapur, 1997; Parr, Byng, Gilpin, & Ireland, 1997). Published accounts of personal experience are more commonly available in the community (e.g., Hewson, 1986; Turnbridge, 1994) but tend to come from small local publishing companies and to disappear from public awareness fairly quickly. The published qualitative research studies that look at lived experience are drawn from personal narratives, yet the reports of these stories run the risk of being transformed into the scientific genre and losing the story (e.g., Crichton-Smith, 2002; Klompas & Ross, 2004; Reid & Button, 1995; Stewart & Richardson, 2004). One of the traps inherent in such collations of stories is that generalizations are drawn and the recognition of individual or alternative responses is lost. For example, contrary to the generalization regarding stroke as a "biographical disruption," the findings of Faircloth and colleagues from the analysis of accounts of 57 older people from different cultural backgrounds, at 6, 12, 18, and 24 months after stroke, suggest that for many, stroke may in fact be part of the biographical flow (Faircloth, Boylstein, Rittman, Young, & Gubrium, 2004). The people interviewed by the investigators associated stroke with the normal illness expectations of aging, or as part of a wider pattern of comorbid illness (such as diabetes), or as consistent with their previous knowledge or experience of stroke. These findings caution against overgeneralization and assumptions in relation to individual responses.

A good example of a scientifically framed research focus that retains the voice of the persons concerned is presented by Reid and Button (1995). These researchers provide an in-depth content analysis of the story of a 13-year-old girl who had been identified as having language and learning disability from the age of 5 years, along with discussion of and comparison with the stories of five learning-disabled peers. Reid and Button argue: "We do not know how *they* understand their problems and needs. We have studied them, planned for them, educated them, and erased them. We have not listened to *their* voices" (Reid & Button, p. 602). As well as providing stretches of the girl's story in relation to particular issues (such as relationships with teachers, friends, and family), the themes arising across all of the students' stories are identified as isolation, victimization, devaluation, and oppression, which are contextualized using excerpts from her story. These researchers frame their research within the critical perspective of Foucault (1965), arguing that learning disability is socially constructed. The identification of students as learning-disabled is linked to normative expectations and framed within a medical paradigm. Reid and Button argue for the importance of listening to (as in "*really* hearing") the themes arising from these stories in order to recognize the need for the development of ways to empower these students to achieve *their* potential.

It cannot be assumed that professionals and clients have similar understandings of either the condition itself or the adequacy of the services provided. For example, Hersh's qualitative research found considerable divergence in the experiences of people with aphasia regarding ending therapy with the

recollections of their clinicians (Hersh, 2001). A fundamental part of listening involves setting up situations in which the experiences and advice of people with communication disability are sought. As an example, the "Way In" project described by Parr and colleagues with people who have aphasia has resulted in the identification of a simple, concrete framework to use in communicating with professionals about how their communication can be improved to assist interaction (Parr, Pound, & Hewitt, 2006). Although training programs for partners of people with communication disability are not new, typically such programs were designed by speech-language pathologists, but increasingly, people with communication disability are being involved in the initial development phase—for example, in the work of Togher and colleagues in developing training for legal and related professionals to interact with users of alternative and augmentative communication (Togher, Balandin, Young, Given, & Canty, 2006).

The other main part of listening involves "really hearing." This skill has been suggested to rely on recognizing the power of the use of metaphorical language (Frank, 1995). Mastergeorge (1999) looked at the use of metaphorical language in relation to communication disorders through the analysis of interviews with 60 families: 37 parents of children with communication disorders; 18 spouses of adults with traumatic brain injury; and 5 adults who stuttered. The analysis identified key metaphors used by these people in their stories—for example, in relation to diagnosis referring to sleep states ("walking into a dream"), barrier structures ("doors closed"), and forces of nature ("we were in rocky waters on a sinking ship"). Such metaphors allow the listener to identify the frames of reference used by the person, thereby offering a medium of communication in framing subsequent discussions and counseling.

Story-telling is part and parcel of every clinical interaction, from the case history to the engagement with the client on a regular basis. The role of story-telling, however, becomes highlighted in the context of group therapy and self-help groups (discussed further later on). For such groups, story-telling takes on the function of what Frank (1995) describes as "bearing witness." Group members introduce themselves in terms of their story ("My name is Joe, and I had a stroke 3 years ago"). Their identity in relation to the group is defined by their illness or disability. This function of groups to shape identity is one of the powerful influences for change but also, at the same time, one of the reasons why some patients prefer individual over group therapy, not wishing to identify "self" with disability. This identification process also raises important questions regarding the notion of recovery: For example, when and how is personal identity further transformed from group membership to community membership? People's stories are dynamic in the sense that as their identity shifts, so too does the story; it is through the constant reiteration of this story that change occurs (that is, the discourse both reflects and shapes change). But individual and group story-telling also is about teaching others, through what Frank describes as the "pedagogy of suffering" (p. 145); this role puts agency back with the person.

When Experts Learn from Patients' Talk

Frank (1995) stresses that the importance of recognizing the reciprocal relationship between the caregiver (including the professional) and the ill person: Both are literally needy, and the recognition of this paradox lays an ethical groundwork for the relationship—that is, an honest recognition of the professional's need to care.

The professional learns from the ill person through hearing the person's testimony, placing the client's meanings alongside professional meanings. For professionals, the ethical challenge, then, is also to reflect on their own stories, their own needs. The professional is changed just as the teller is changing through the reiteration of the story. As Pound suggests, such learning is challenging: "Professional culture has little space for personal becoming. Young doctors are not trained to think of the careers ahead of them as trajectories of their own moral development, which is one reason why they have trouble with an expanded notion of service" (Pound, 2004, p. 159).

Few published stories of speech-language pathologists' "lessons learned" are available (Hinckley, 2007) and, so it is interesting to look more closely at four such stories recently told by experts in the field of aphasiology (Duchan & Byng, 2004).

One such expert, Carol Pound, talks of her "journey," seeing a transition from chaos, a change from restitution to quest (Pound, 2004). From her personal experience as a patient, she distills lessons of the importance of control and the recognition of expertise (by self and others) in the lived experience of the condition. Pound writes the type of quest narrative that falls within Frank's description of *manifesto* in the sense of lessons learned now being taught as suggestions for change—even though she explicitly balances these suggestions for change with recognition of alternative viewpoints.

For Jon Lyon (2004), the lessons are learned both directly and indirectly from people with aphasia. From a client he considered to be "more a mentor than a client" (p. 78), Lyon learned the importance of activities that allow being "in the moment." Indirectly, from other experiences over the years, he learned the importance of choosing targets that allow for some degree of "ease" or automaticity to be gained in their use, through selecting goals that fit in with what the person can do and that fit within the broader script of their life. The narrative of the journey that Lyon has taken over 30 years in working with aphasia largely takes the form of a memoir—events and stages, interspersed with key moments of insight.

For Claire Penn (2004), the personal journey is not so much about what she should or should not be doing in aphasia therapy: From the outset, she responded to the wider life needs of the person with aphasia (for example, as a student, she abandoned a more formal approach and instead interacted through playing cards with a patient whose language she did not share). Rather, her struggle is with the legitimacy of such responses. She asked herself repeatedly: If this is what I am doing, then am I or should I be a speech pathologist? This issue became most critical when a long-standing "successful" client committed suicide (Penn, 1993). Her account of therapy with her client Valerie Rosen-

berg compares her own experience with Valerie's account of the stages of therapy, largely as an example of both client-led therapy and the boundaries of her role (time-limited by stages in recovery and role-limited through identification of the need for counseling support as informed by her previous experience). Penn learned from her wider cultural experience the central importance of her role as an aphasia therapist " . . . to fight tooth and nail amidst changing health policy and the redistribution of resources" (p. 86), arguing for advocacy.

Audrey Holland and Amy Ramage's account of "learning from Roger Ross" explicitly notes that this close personal and professional relationship with their client Roger Ross both reinforced the clinicians' views and understandings of therapy, but "others he helped us develop" (Holland & Ramage, 2004, p. 118). These workers report their personal lessons as learning that "we are not experts in anyone's aphasia," and that "often, in clinical interactions with aphasic persons, the behavior that needs to be changed is our own" (p. 128). Like Lyons, Pound, and Penn, they note the evolving process of coming to live with aphasia, not just for the person with aphasia but for themselves professionally.

Frank (1995) argues that the postmodern perspective is not an abnegation of moral responsibility through the movement away from seeking absolute truths of a situation but is instead fundamentally ethical in that this perspective highlights the need for individual responsibility in the search for meaning. In this situation of seeking to understand the perspectives of people with communication disorders, a postmodern approach to intervention is about "hearing" the person's search for meaning as much as it is about providing treatments. This hearing is not just about listening to the person talk—as Frank points out, stories are enacted as well as told, so it also is about being fully present as the person enacts his or her story and finds meaning for the lived experience. Frank suggests that this hearing is each person's ethical responsibility, whether or not this is seen as part of the scope of professional practice. He does note personal and professional limits, however, in reminding readers that even the Good Samaritan paid someone else to take care of the man found beside the road. Frank is suggesting that a holistic view of professional responsibility for services is not a burden in the sense that professionals are responsible for everything about everyone: From a postmodern perspective, the professional is no longer a "hero," nor are patients expected to be Phoenix-like, reborn from the conflagration of their disability without the grief from memories of their former lives (Frank, 2000, p.136). Choices are available, and people have their own meanings to create from their experiences. The evolution of these meanings is mediated through the interactions between professionals and their clients, between professionals and the system, and between clients and the institutions on which they rely.

Collaboration and Partnership

Collaboration and partnership approaches often meet with resistance, either overtly or more often through passive resistance, from professionals. Passive resistance probably is the most potent force against the achievement of collaboration, because lip service is paid to the benefits of partnership, yet nothing fundamentally changes in practice. Resistance often takes the form of arguments that current best practice already involves taking patients' needs into account and hence already represents a partnership. The question arises, then, of what underlies such resistance.

As discussed by Veatch in relation to the medical profession, today the consumer is well informed and supported through advocacy groups, and the physician can feel loss of control and autonomy in professional practice (Veatch, 2000). Resistance to partnership approaches, however, should not be oversimplified as presenting threats to power and status. In the Western culture of individualism, the person seeks the service without a view to the collective good—that is, the priorities for service provision for the population as a whole. So when services are not available, then pressure is put on the professional—but the professional may be more conscious of total caseload or health and education service demands. Veatch argues that the clinician is caught in an ethical dilemma: Strictly speaking, the clinician cannot know the best course to follow medically (because of the limits of evidence in any area), nor can the clinician know what is the best course to follow holistically (because of the limits of knowing what is best for another person). Veatch also argues, however, that the clinician cannot abnegate responsibility for decisions either, noting wryly the absurd consequences of a shift from the Hippocratic oath to essentially its opposite: "Warning all ye who enter here. I have been asked by society to abandon you at the margin and serve society as its cost-containment agent" (p. 718). In view of the limits of the clinician's knowing, the most fundamental aspect of collaboration and partnership in decisions about service provision comes down to harnessing the patient's ability to "know best," and this entails empowerment, discussed next.

Empowerment and Self-Help Groups: Who's the Expert?

The term *empowerment* raises multiple issues both in terms of the type of power evoked and the relationships conjured up by the prefix. Types of power usually are thought of as involving legitimate (institutional) power (such as that of an employer or the police), the power of coercive force (e.g., physical), the power of rewards or incentives (and rewards withheld, such as payment), and the power of influence (e.g., persuasion). The exertion of power results in an effect on someone else, so power is not so much a state as an action. The types of power that affect professionals' lives typically involve all of the aforementioned except coercive force, but the lives of patients may be affected by all types of power. *Em*powerment is the process whereby individual people or groups are provided with the tools (knowledge, skills, and attitudes) that will enable them to influence the other people, agencies, and institutions that affect their lives. Thus, the type of power involved here is that of influence, although the goal of such influence is to harness other powerful processes that will improve services (for example, legislation). One of the paradoxes inherent in empowerment is that power is being "given" or transferred from the powerful to the powerless, which is itself is a form of benevolent paternalism, while at the same time the ideology of empowerment is about recognition of rights to autonomy and self-determination.

Empowerment is not without its detractors. According to Wolfensberger, a prominent proponent of advocacy, the ideology of empowerment assumes that autonomy and self-determination are "good"—of value to the person (Wolfensberger, 2003b). This author argues that the ideology of empowerment has a religion-like quality in that it is a value (not empirical), and that self-determination may not be always in the best interests of the person with disability. For example, a person may have autonomy to choose but little to choose from, or problems can arise if the person who is not competent in decision-making is "given" self-determination.

As previously discussed, considerable power inheres within group interactions for change and adjustment to disability, and such processes can take place within therapy groups (Elman, 2006), as well as self-help groups. When such groups turn their attention to influencing the wider community (such as through their stories and lessons to pass on to professionals and the public), then processes of empowerment are at work both for persons within the group and for the group itself.

The power of influence from peers is the main source of explanation for why self-help groups are empowering. This sort of *referent* power has been compared with that of *expert* power in a study that included 156 members of mental health self-help groups (Salem, Reischl, Gallacher, & Randall, 2000).

Not unexpectedly, greater referent power was ascribed to members, and greater expert power was ascribed both to leaders and more so to professionals. Of interest, the amount of perceived helpfulness of the group was predicted by higher expert power, although when referent power was high, expert power ceased to be predictive of perceived usefulness.

The dangers of the movement toward service provision via self-help groups need to be recognized. In a personal account of mental health services, Gibson-Leek (2003) argues that proliferation of self-help services are a cheap way for governments to look as though they are fulfilling the need for community-based services, but such services can be dangerous to consumers, for example, when run by "controlling" persons without adequate training and who are not governed by professional principles. Gibson-Leek also argues against the development of professional clients who are paid for their services, for example, to sit on advocacy panels, rejecting their right to speak on the behalf of others.

This personal account accords with some of the issues raised in the discussion of the "Expert Patient" program in the United Kingdom (Wilson, 2001), which was designed as an attempt to deal with chronic illness in a more holistic way. Basically, the program involved identifying the patient with chronic illness as the "expert" by virtue of personal experience and moved the emphasis to self-management strategies. Wilson notes that problems arise from a false shift of power—for example, the power to deem what may be appropriate self-management still rests with medical professional perspective,

with movements toward alternative treatments rejected. Expert patients are expected to self-manage their conditions, but only in the "right" way. When the patient fails to adopt "approved" self-management strategies (such as eating healthily or stopping smoking), then the system opens the possibility of a "blame the patient" philosophy, with potential use of power to apply sanctions (such as withholding services). From a foucauldian perspective (Foucault, 1973), the system exerts "pastoral power" in that the patient's lifestyle becomes open to surveillance and judgment. Self-management is seen as potentially marginalizing chronic illness (away from the higher funding associated with technical medicine), yet at the same time as threatening to professionals in possibly opening up demands for support services that are not available. In other words, the resultant power tensions here are complex, and realizing the benefits of empowerment requires careful consideration of the ethical issues involved.

The involvement of speech-language pathologists with self-help groups has tended on the whole to reflect a strong demarcation between professional and client. Examples of the tensions that arise between professionals and members of self-help groups are evident in the area of stuttering. In a study of the perceived benefits of membership in the National Stuttering Association (NSA), findings from a questionnaire given to 71 adults diagnosed with this disorder indicated that the partnership between professional speech-language pathologists and self-help groups was limited (Yaruss et al., 2002). According to this study, although an increasing number of professionals are becoming

NSA members, only a small proportion (9 of 71) of the adult clients surveyed indicated that they had been encouraged to join by speech-language pathologists, although 16 were in treatment at the time they first attended.

Provocatively, Onslow and Costa argued that the role of self-help groups with regard to the maintenance phase of behavioral management programs for stuttering fell outside the expertise of self-help groups, although these investigators acknowledged the importance of such groups for more general support (Onslow & Costa, 1989). In a spirited response, a leading figure within the self-help association for people who stutter in Australia (SpeakEasy) argued that self-help groups were filling an important role in service provision, through the practice opportunities for speech restructuring techniques and support for maintenance of fluency (Bartley, 1990). The arguments put forward by Bartley called forth a further response from Beilby, another speech-language pathologist, reacting strongly against implications of any inadequacies in professional services that self-help groups could be seen as addressing (Beilby, 1991). This debate essentially centered on divergent notions of what constitutes expertise, with the self-help group arguing for lived experience of stuttering management techniques as transferable expertise and the professionals arguing for the primacy of educational and professional experience of stuttering management techniques as the sole basis for transferable expertise. To pit these views against each other fails to recognize the benefits of partnership. In the words of one person with a communication disorder recounting his experience, "The supporting nature of speech therapy and self-help group

is beyond price. . . . To be able to speak from direct experience is crucial" (Stewart & Richardson, 2004, p. 102).

The role of persons with communication disorders and their caregivers with regard to influencing service provision has been little explored. Kamhi (1999) suggests that parents of children with communication disorders are one source of influence on therapists' use of therapy approaches. Beyond this role of influence, Pound describes the work being done through the Connect program in the United Kingdom in which direct services are provided by people with aphasia in training conversation skills of volunteers working in the program, such as providing feedback to shape supportive communication strategies (Pound, 2004) .

The goal of empowerment usually is to gain more services, but Kagan and Duchan (2004) suggest that the consumer perspective also is needed to evaluate services. These researchers note that typically what is being evaluated and the method of evaluation used are chosen by the professionals, even when consumer satisfaction, communicative effectiveness, and quality of life questionnaires, for example, are used as part of the evaluation process. Kagan and Duchan ask the question "Who is the expert?" with regard to evaluating. In a person-centered approach, they argue, consumers are the experts in whether they got what they wanted and are the experts to be consulted in devising ways to measure this. Although communication challenges remain to be overcome in involving people with communication difficulties in evaluative processes, these investigators' report on findings from qualitative research using in-depth interview methods found important differences in what to measure, with talking but also personal or emotional and wider environmental or life participation issues seen as important, with less concern with clinical service matters.

Advocacy (and the Perils of Expertise)

Advocacy essentially means speaking on another's behalf, but as Wolfensberger (2003a) points out, advocacy goes beyond the typical responsibilities of a service provider. In fact, the advocacy role potentially places the clinician in a position of conflict of interest: Responsibilities are owed to both the patient and the employing institution, for example, as well as to the standards and prevailing paradigms of the profession. Such conflicts of interest arise for professionals working outside clinical roles. Munger (2000) discusses the conflicts of interest for economic policy analysts, noting the need to recognize the different weights and different values on key issues and ways forward for those affected by advocacy, those employing the expert, and the experts' professional precepts. From the perspective of the person with a communication disorder, it may be seen that more services—say, home-based—are needed, but from the professional perspective, it may be considered that more research still needs to be done to know what sort of services work best in this service delivery model (most research having been done in clinical settings), and from the employer's perspective, it may be recognized that limits exist with regard to funding, time, or staffing resources to provide these services. How, then, do these pressures affect the expert's ability to provide independent advocacy, and what can be done about the inherent conflicts?

In their discussion of the multiple roles played by experts in class action cases advocating for mental health services, Hoge and colleagues note that the problems arise when conflicts of interest are not acknowledged (Hoge, Tebes, Davidson, & Griffith, 2002). For example, when an expert witness is retained by one or other side in the adversarial system, but then moves to act as a consulting expert to the service, or is appointed by the court to monitor actions taken. Although impartiality is assumed (as a professional precept), the group process of being part of a particular team putting forward a particular view influences the advocacy. Indeed, the decision to take on the role of advocate implies support for a particular point of view and thus represents an opinion, no matter how evidence-based such an opinion or judgment may be.

Advocacy for persons with communication disorders within speech-language pathology practice is likely to be more widespread than is currently acknowledged. As discussed in Chapter 3, in a study that looked at the reports by eight speech-language pathologists of 15 critical incidents involving legal decision-making in working with people with aphasia, seven participants identified that they had taken advocacy roles with patients in the sense of speaking on their behalf in family and case conferences (Duffield, Ferguson, & Worrall, 2007; Ferguson et al., 2004).

Advocacy for services is seen to fall within the scope of practice of speech-language pathologists (see Chapter 1). Sarno argues that advocacy is particularly important in speech-language pathology because of the invisibility of communication disorders. She notes the lack of public awareness about aphasia, for example, despite its high prevalence, and argues that speech-language pathologists have a moral responsibility for advocacy (Sarno, 2004). But to what extent is such advocacy a matter of self-interest (generating more services to be provided by speech-language pathologists), and to what extent does advocacy reflect the need for the types of services that will benefit people with communication disorders? Increasing attention is being paid to the kind of research that enables a view of needed services from a consumer perspective (Kagan & Duchan, 2004; Parr & Byng, 2000; Worrall et al., 2006). Interviews, conducted either face to face or by telephone, and focus groups provide accessible methodologies that can be used by clinical services to explore local population needs (Machin, Ferguson, Alston, & Laney, 2004; O'Neill, Machin, Ferguson, Laney, & Alston, 2007). On a bigger scale, Kagan and LeBlanc (2002) have described a "nuts and bolts" model for how professionals work to advocate for improvement of services, listing important strategies as including partnership with other professionals, and working from already-known concepts of decision-makers to forge the links from physical to communication needs (as in the use of the metaphor "communication ramps" needed for assisting communication).

One way out of the dilemma of benevolently assuming the needs of others is the recognition of the important role of *self-advocacy*. This concept is linked inextricably with empowerment: The professional works with the person with a communication disorder so that the person is able to speak on his or her own behalf—as Pound describes it, "giving people with aphasia and others the tools to access services, complain about service gaps, expect flexible and multifaceted support opportunities" (Pound, 2004, p. 45). Self-advocacy requires the provision of accessible information about rights, systems, and processes. The provision of this information brings attention back to the role of discourse in empowerment. The kinds of services speech-language pathologists discuss with clients, as well as the manner in which such information is presented, will shape clients' access to knowledge. This knowledge will allow persons with communication disorders to make the choices they need regarding their role in shaping the services provided to them and to others.

References

Bartley, P. (1990). Ivory towers and glass houses: Does the dog have fleas? The real story on the role and purpose of stutterers' self-help groups in Australia. *Australian Journal of Human Communication Disorders, 18*(1), 79–88.

Barton, E. L. (1999). The social work of diagnosis: Evidence for judgments of competence and incompetence. In D. Kovarsky, J. F. Duchan, & M. Maxwell (Eds.), *Constructing (in)competence: Disabling evaluations in clinical and social interaction* (pp. 257–288). Mahwah, NJ: Lawrence Erlbaum Associates.

Beilby, J. (1991). Letter to the editor. *Australian Journal of Human Communication Disorders, 19*(1), 102.

Crichton-Smith, I. (2002). Communicating in the real world: Accounts from people who stammer. *Journal of Fluency Disorders, 27,* 333–352.

Duchan, J., & Byng, S. (2004). *Challenging aphasia therapies*. Hove, UK: Psychology Press.

Duffield, G., Ferguson, A., & Worrall, L. (2007). *Legal issues and aphasia: Critical incidents for speech pathologists*. Paper presented at the Speech Pathology Association of Australia national conference, Sydney, May 27–31.

Elman, R. J. (2006). *Group treatment of neurogenic communication disorders: The expert clinician's approach*. San Diego, CA: Plural.

Faircloth, C. A., Boylstein, C., Rittman, M., Young, M. E., & Gubrium, J. (2004). Sudden illness and biographical flow in narratives of stroke recovery. *Sociology of Health & Illness, 26*(2), 242–261.

Ferguson, A., Worrall, L., McPhee, J., Buskell, R., Armstrong, E., & Togher, L. (2004). *Autonomy in life decisions for people with aphasia: Issues for speech pathologists*. Paper presented at the 26th World Congress of the International Association of Logopedics & Phoniatrics, Brisbane, Australia, Aug. 29–Sept. 2.

Foucault, M. (1965). *Madness and civilization: A history of insanity in the Age of Reason* (R. Howard, Trans.). London: Tavistock.

Foucault, M. (1973). *The birth of the clinic: An archaeology of medical perception* (A. M. Sheridan Smith, Trans.). New York: Vintage Books.

Frank, A. W. (1995). *The wounded storyteller: Body, illness, and ethics*. Chicago: University of Chicago Press.

Gibson-Leek, M. (2003). Personal Account: Client versus client. *Psychiatric Services, 54*(8), 1101–1102.

Goffman, E. (1971). *Relations in public*. Harmondsworth, UK: Penguin.

Goffman, E. (1990). *Stigma: Notes on the management of spoiled identity*. London: Penguin Books.

Hersh, D. (2001). Experiences of ending aphasia therapy. *International Journal of Language & Communication Disorders, 36*(Suppl.), 80–85.

Hewson, L. (1986). *When half is whole: My recovery from stroke*. Blackburn, Victoria, Australia: Collins Dove.

Hinckley, J. J. (2007). *Narrative-based practice in speech-language pathology*. San Diego, CA: Plural Publishing.

Hoge, M. A., Tebes, J. K., Davidson, L., & Griffith, E. E. H. (2002). The roles of behavioral health professionals in class action litigation. *Journal of the American Academy of Psychiatry & the Law, 30*(1), 49–58.

Holland, A. L., & Ramage, A. E. (2004). Learning from Roger Ross: A clinical journey. In J. F. Duchan & S. Byng (Eds.), *Challenging aphasia therapies: Broadening the discourse and extending the boundaries* (pp. 118–129). Hove, UK: Psychology Press.

Kagan, A., & Duchan, J. F. (2004). Consumers' views of what makes therapy worthwhile. In J. F. Duchan & S. Byng (Eds.), *Challenging aphasia therapies: Broadening the discourse and extending the boundaries* (pp. 158–172). Hove, UK: Psychology Press.

Kagan, A., & LeBlanc, K. (2002). Motivating for infrastructure change: Toward a communicatively accessible, participation-based stroke care system for all those affected by aphasia. *Journal of Communication Disorders, 35*, 153–169.

Kamhi, A. G. (1999). To use or not to use: Factors that influence the selection of new treatment approaches. *Language, Speech, and Hearing Services in Schools, 30*(1), 92–98.

Kapur, N. (Ed.). (1997). *Injured brains of medical minds: Views from within*. Oxford: Oxford University Press.

Klompas, M., & Ross, E. (2004). Life experiences of people who stutter, and the perceived impact of stuttering on quality of life: Personal accounts of South African individuals. *Journal of Fluency Disorders, 29*, 275–305.

Law, J., Bunning, K., Byng, S., Farrelly, S., & Heyman, B. (2005). Making sense in primary care: Levelling the playing field for people with communication difficulties. *Disability & Society*, 20(2), 169–184.

Lubkin, I. M., & Larsen, P. D. (2006). *Chronic illness: Impact and interventions* (6th ed.). Boston: Jones and Bartlett.

Lyon, J. (2004). Evolving treatment methods for coping with aphasia approaches that make a difference in everyday life. In J. F. Duchan (Ed.), *Challenging aphasia therapies: Broadening the discourse and extending the boundaries* (pp. 54–82). Hove, UK: Psychology Press.

Machin, P., Ferguson, A., Alston, M., & Laney, G. (2004). *On-going support for people with aphasia: Finding out the needs.* Paper presented at the 26th World Congress of the International Association of Logopedics and Phoniatrics, Brisbane, Australia, Aug. 29–Sept. 2.

Mackay, R. (2003). "Tell them who I was" [1]: The social construction of aphasia. *Disability & Society*, 18(6), 811–826.

Mastergeorge, A. M. (1999). Revelations of family perceptions of diagnosis and disorder through metaphor (ch.11). In D. Kovarsky, J. F. Duchan, & M. Maxwell (Eds.), *Constructing (in)competence: Disabling evaluations in clinical and social interaction* (pp. 245–256). Mahwah, NJ: Lawrence Erlbaum Associates.

Munger, M. C. (2000). Experts and "advocacy": The limits of policy analysis. In *Analyzing policy: Choices, conflicts, and practices* (pp. 134–161). New York: W. W. Norton.

O'Neill, I., Machin, P., Ferguson, A., Laney, G., & Alston, M. (2007). *Quality of life in individuals with aphasia: Use of a mixed methods approach.* Paper presented at the Speech Pathology Australia national conference, Sydney, May 27–31.

Onslow, M., & Costa, L. (1989). When the tail begins to wag the dog: Some views on the relationship between speech pathologists and self-help groups in the management of stuttering. *Australian Journal of Human Communication Disorders*, 17(2), 77–86.

Parr, S., Byng, S., Gilpin, S., & Ireland, C. (1997). *Talking about aphasia.* Buckingham, UK: Open University Press.

Parr, S., & Byng, S. C. (2000). Perspectives and priorities: Accessing user views in functional communication assessment. In L. E. Worrall & C. M. Frattali (Eds.), *Neurogenic communication disorders: A functional approach* (pp. 55–66). New York: Thieme.

Parr, S., Pound, C., & Hewitt, A. (2006). Communication access to health and social services. *Topics in Language Disorders*, 26(3), 189–198.

Penn, C. (1993). Aphasia therapy in South Africa: Some pragmatic and personal perspectives. In A. Holland & M. M. Forbes (Eds.), *Aphasia treatment: World perspectives.* San Diego, CA: Singular.

Penn, C. (2004). Context, culture, and conversation. In J. F. Duchan & S. Byng (Eds.), *Challenging aphasia therapies: Broadening the discourse and extending the boundaries* (pp. 83–100). Hove, UK: Psychology Press.

Pound, C. (2004). Dare to be different: The person and the practice. In J. F. Duchan (Ed.), *Challenging aphasia therapies: Broadening the discourse and extending the boundaries* (pp. 32–53). Hove, UK: Psychology Press.

Reid, D. K., & Button, L. G. (1995). Anna's story: Narratives of personal experience about being labeled learning disabled. *Journal of Learning Disabilities*, 28(10), 602–614.

Salem, D. A., Reischl, T. M., Gallacher, F., & Randall, K. W. (2000). The role of referent and expert power in mutual help. *American Journal of Community Psychology*, 28(3), 303–324.

Sarno, M. T. (2004). Aphasia therapies: Historical perspectives and moral imperatives. In J. F. Duchan & S. Byng (Eds.), *Challenging aphasia therapies: Broadening the discourse and extending the boundaries* (pp. 19–31). Hove, UK: Psychology Press.

Stewart, T., & Richardson, G. (2004). A qualitative study of therapeutic effect from a user's perspective. *Journal of Fluency Disorders*, 29, 95–108.

Togher, L., Balandin, S., Young, K., Given, F., & Canty, M. (2006). Development of a communication training program to improve access to legal services for people with complex communication needs. *Topics in Language Disorders*, 26(3), 199–209.

Turnbridge, N. (1994). *The stutterer's survival guide*. Sydney: Addison-Wesley.

Veatch, R. M. (2000). Doctor does not know best: Why in the new century physicians must stop trying to benefit patients. *Journal of Medicine and Philosophy*, 25(6), 701–721.

Wilson, P. M. (2001). A policy analysis of the Expert Patient in the United Kingdom: Self-care as an expression of pastoral power? *Health & Social Care in the Community*, 9(3), 134–142.

Wolfensberger, W. (2003a). Advocacy. In D. G. Race (Ed.), *Leadership and change in human services: Selected readings from Wolf Wolfensberger* (pp. 119–149). London: Routledge.

Wolfensberger, W. (2003b). Social role valorization. In D. G. Race (Ed.), *Leadership and change in human services: Selected readings from Wolf Wolfensberger* (pp. 80–118). London: Routledge.

Worrall, L. (2000). The influence of professional values on the functional communication approach in aphasia. In L. E. Worrall & C. M. Frattali (Eds.), *Neurogenic communication disorders: A functional approach* (pp. 191–205). New York: Thieme.

Worrall, L. (2006). Professionalism and functional outcomes. *Journal of Communication Disorders*, 39, 320–327.

Worrall, L., Davidson, B., Hersh, D., Howe, T., Ferguson, A., & Sherratt, S. (2006). *What people with aphasia want: Toward person-centred goal-setting in aphasia rehabilitation*. Research in progress. Unpublished manuscript.

Yaruss, J. S., Quesal, R. W., Reeves, L., Molt, L. F., Kluetz, B., Caruso, A. J., et al. (2002). Speech treatment and support group experiences of people who participate in the National Stuttering Association. *Journal of Fluency Disorders*, 27, 115–134.

5

Working Collaboratively: Discourse Involves Multiple Parties

In an ideal world, interdisciplinary teams work together smoothly to provide intervention, but in reality, communication processes present major challenges to the provision of health care. Multiple terms have proliferated to describe the many ways in which professionals work together: interdisciplinary, multidisciplinary, transdisciplinary, interprofessional. In this chapter, the term *multidisciplinary* is reserved for situations in which professionals from specific disciplines retain their professional identities, contributing discipline-specific knowledge or skills to a situation. The term *transdisciplinary* is used to refer to situations in which professions adopt and integrate the knowledge and skills of other disciplines within shared practice. The terms *interdisciplinary* and *interprofessional* are used somewhat interchangeably to refer generically to situations in which professionals from different disciplines work together, although the term *interprofessional* is favored when the discus-

sion is about aspects of professional practice, rather than aspects related to the theoretical or empirical frameworks informing the discipline. Also, the terms *collaboration* and *partnership*, used widely in the literature, are used synonymously in this chapter.

Many aspects of working collaboratively have been recognized, but collaborative work is mediated primarily through discourse. Roberts and Sarangi identify three main discourses in which professionals are involved: personal discourse (describing their own experiences), professional discourse (the discourse needed to carry out their professional roles), and institutional discourse (the discourse that describes and accounts for professional discourse) (Roberts & Sarangi, 2003). Chapter 1 of this book explored some of the aspects of institutional discourse (through examination of documents describing scope of practice), and Chapter 4 looked at some of the published material on discourse describing

the personal experiences of professionals. This chapter focuses on professional discourse and, in particular, on
the discourse required by professionals
when working together.

Speaking the Same Language

One of the most apparent areas of
difficulty that arises in the discourse
between members of different professional groups is the difficulty with terminology (Walsh, 2005). Even the terms
used to describe the profession itself
are not unproblematic. For example,
Ukrainetz and Fresquez (2003) found
that speech-language pathologists working in schools described themselves as
"speech teachers" with their school
students, and as either "speech therapists" or "speech pathologists" when
talking with teachers. Of interest, one
participant described her reluctance to
use the term "speech-language pathologist" with reference to the sociocultural
implications of increasing the perceived
status gap between herself and teachers
(Ukrainetz & Fresquez, p. 288). Within
the profession of speech-language
pathology itself, considerable debate
around terminology remains, extending beyond the trivial. For example,
debates surrounding the use of such
terms as *specific language impairment*,
developmental verbal dyspraxia, and *cluttering* are not reducible to debates
about lists of symptoms that are to be
considered fundamental to the application of the labels. Instead, these debates
center on the extent of shared understanding of the fundamental nature of
the difficulties captured by these terms.

For example, how "specific" is *specific
language impairment*? Does the presence
of other cognitive difficulties mean that
the nature of the type of language problem observed is any different (Plante,
1998)? As another example, is there a
qualitative difference in the types of
difficulties seen in children with severe
phonological disorder compared with
those seen in developmental verbal
dyspraxia, and if (as some researchers
argue) the differences observed point
to the presence of neurological impairment, then is the presence of neurological symptoms sufficient to clearly
differentiate the two? This debate has
resulted in the proposal to use *childhood
apraxia of speech* instead of the now
muddied term *developmental verbal dyspraxia of speech* (Forrest, 2003). If experienced clinicians are able to "know
cluttering when they hear it," does it
matter that checklists of diagnostic
symptoms for stuttering, prosodic and
articulatory disorders, and cluttering
fail to clearly delineate the category of
"cluttering"? (St. Louis, Raphael, Myers,
& Bakker, 2003). Such terminological
debates are important to the profession
and are likely to continue, despite
repeated calls for consistency of use of
terms, because terms and meanings
undergo change over time, as is the
way of all language use, reflecting
shifts in the culture of speech-language
pathology. The debates themselves,
however, are important to the profession, because such debates reflect the
sharing and growth of understandings of
communication disorders among members of the professional community.
Despite inconsistencies and differences
in use of terms, shared understandings
are likely to be sufficient to prevent
serious misunderstandings between

people. For example, the historical term "developmental aphasia" is no longer used but is still available in the shared consciousness of the profession, allowing access to historical understandings of child language disorders (Eadie, 2005; Kamhi, 1998).

More difficulties with terminology arise in interprofessional contexts for which shared understandings have not emerged. In general, such interprofessional misunderstandings are described in terms of the uses and abuses of jargon that is specific to the particular profession. For example, if a speech-language pathologist uses a profession-specific term such as *phonological input lexicon*, or a linguistic term such as *left embedding*, then it is only reasonable that a doctor, nurse, or teacher would not understand what is meant. In such situations, however, it is clear to listeners or readers that they have not understood, and this awareness provides the potential trigger for seeking clarification.

More fundamental misunderstandings can arise when each person is assuming that the other is using terms in the same way, without either party being aware of the difficulty. Such problems arise when everyday words are used by one profession in very specific ways. For example, the term *comprehension* is used very narrowly in speech-language pathology to relate to comprehension of written or spoken language that is separable from other cognitive skills such as memory or executive judgment and decision-making, whereas in the general community, *comprehension* typically embraces all such meanings. Both the adoption of novel jargon and the narrowing of meaning of everyday terms to convey specific profession-related meanings

are common to every social grouping within a community. The idiosyncratic sets of terms and meanings in different health and education disciplines, for example, differ not only from each other but also from the discourse of the administrative organization, so that words such as "report to" may imply "keep informed" to a clinician but "be directly supervised" to an administrator (Schroeder et al., 1999). Such misunderstandings can be expected in all types of interprofessional discourse.

A good example of problems with terminology was highlighted in the findings of research on teachers' awareness of language impairment (Webb, 2007). Webb used a questionnaire to find out more about the understanding of 215 teachers with regard to a number of aspects of matters related to speech-language pathology (for the 6- to 12-year-old age group). In their responses to the questionnaire, teachers used "speech" and "language" interchangeably (pp.157–158). Similar terminology issues were reported by Ukrainetz and Fresquez (2003) in their qualitative study of such usages by 5 speech-language pathologists and 15 teachers. The term *language* appeared to be a general umbrella term for teachers in their study, in comparison with the very specific aspects of language (such as syntax and semantics) that fell within the use of this term for the speech-language pathologists. Such terminology issues present a significant barrier to collaborative approaches widely held to be of value in this area, as discussed by Tollerfield (2003), who similarly found that speech-language pathologists working with teachers needed to explain such terms as "receptive" and "expressive." From an analysis of 50 in-depth interviews with early childhood teachers, Mroz (2006) reports that the identification of children with communication disorders was a major concern to teachers, and the suggested need for training in this area would rely heavily on clear description and definition.

Although use of terminology points toward the important role of understanding discourse in interprofessional interaction, in one sense terminology issues are relatively straightforward to address—through awareness, and with an attitude of responsiveness and mutual respect in seeking clarification. Terminology, however, is just one small part of the wider complexities in interprofessional discourse.

Working Together

Working together in collaborative partnerships can involve many different ways of relating, which fall somewhere along a continuum of independence to interdependence. For example, referral from one professional to another leaves both professionals working very separately, yet each relies on the other for some aspect of service delivery. Somewhere toward the middle of this continuum would fall the type of collaboration in which the speech-language pathologist works alongside another professional, for example, in a multidisciplinary team. Toward closer interdependence falls the type of partnership in which the professionals are involved in simultaneous service provision to the client.

One of the most tightly interdependent working relationships between a speech-language pathologist and another professional occurs in work with an interpreter in either the assessment or the treatment of a client, in that the speech-language pathologist is unable to assess the client without the mediation of the interpreter—for example, when the client speaks another spoken or signed language (Isaac, 2001; Seal, 2000). The complexity of the discourse in interpreter-mediated sessions is illustrated in Examples 5–1 and 5–2.

Example 5–1 is drawn from the research of Roger (2003) into interpreter-mediated assessment of people with aphasia. In this example, the speech-language pathologist is trying to assess a patient with a tentative diagnosis of aphasia following stroke, and the interpreter is attempting to interpret (into Tagalog) as the speech-language pathologist administers the repetition task from the Western Aphasia Battery (Kertesz, 1982, 2006). On coming to the item "The pastry cook was elated," the interpreter has been uncertain as to how to interpret "elated." Perhaps deciding that an online discussion regarding items of similar co-articulatory complexity was not possible at that moment, the speech-language pathologist instead asks the interpreter to find a word of roughly equivalent meaning. This moment involves a shift in what Goffman (1974) describes as a "frame," in that the culturally framed role of "interpreter" has shifted—now the interpreter is deciding on and providing stimuli, rather than straightforward interpreting. A second frame shift occurs at utterance 4, when the speech-language pathologist inquires about the clarity of the patient's repetition attempt—here again, the interpreter's role shifts again from interpreting to evaluating. This type of frame shift

---

Example 5–1
Interpreter-Mediated Assessment

(*Key:* I, interpreter; P, patient; S, speech-language pathologist; =, simultaneous talk.)

1 S: Just say "happy" . . . "happy"'s fine . . . instead of "elated," just say "happy."

2 I: *Ang tagapagluto ay masaya.*

3 P: *Ang tag-pagluto masaya.*

4 S: Clear?

5 I: Ah . . . no . . . a bit . . . not clear . . . *tagapagluto* . . . [slowly to P] *ang tagapagluto ay masaya.*

6 P: *Ang tagipagluto masaya.*

7 S: Better that time . . . or not?

8 I: No . . . no . . . I mean . . . um . . . like . . . It's a bit . . . not . . . ah . . . there is like a . . .

9 S: Okay, this . . . how does it sound different?

10 I: No, it's not different but ah . . . you know it's just like . . . ah . . . like stuttering . . . something like that.

Reproduced with permission of the author from: Roger, P. (2003). *Linguistic diversity and the assessment of aphasia.* Unpublished PhD thesis, University of Sydney, Sydney, Australia.

---

is extremely common in interpreter-mediated speech pathology sessions and causes considerable tension and concern for interpreters, because it challenges their professional precepts regarding the importance of *not* judging (Ferguson, Candlin, Armstrong, Isaac, & Roger, 2005; Isaac, Roger, Candlin, Ferguson, & Armstrong, 2004). This moment in the interaction also represents what Goffman describes as a shift in "footing" (Goffman, 1981, p. 124) within the frame, in that here the speech-language pathologist and the interpreter align, aside from the patient, to consult regarding the clarity of the patient's attempt. This footing shift recurs at utterance 7, and in utter-

ance 8, the interpreter can be seen to be displaying a high degree of uncertainty in her response, through discourse markers of hesitancy, and considerable modulation (for example, "it's *a bit* like," "*just* like"). This display of uncertainty signals (whether consciously or unconsciously) that the interpreter is being asked to step outside what Goffman (1974) describes as the "frame space"—that is, the interpreter is being asked to step outside the usual role of an interpreter. The speech-language pathologist in utterance 9 seeks what amounts to a metatextual analysis ("how does it sound different?") as she tries to identify what it is that was different in the patient's repetition (phonology or grammar); this relates to the speech-language pathologist's main agenda, that is, the textual analysis of the patient's utterances. Such meta-textual analysis, however, is well beyond the cultural frame for the interpreter's role. Of note, this interaction is taking place in front of the patient; thus, in line with Goffman's (1974) notions of the "participation framework," the patient is the "audience" as well as the "object" under discussion, so in analyzing this discourse, it needs to be considered whether the choice of words and wordings reflect some adjustment for this audience. For example, noticeably absent are evaluative words such as *wrong* or *error*, with words such as "clear," "not clear," "better," "different," and "not different" being used instead.

From the perspective of the speech-language pathologist, the frame shifts and shifts of footing within the frames in such interactions may be invisible. For the speech-language pathologist, all interactions with the client would involve a "meta-frame," in that the speech-language pathologist is engaging with the client in conversational or testing interactions while simultaneously evaluating the content and form of the language and the interaction itself. The speech-language pathologist's role involves continual adjustments to his or her own contributions to the interaction specifically designed to elicit types of language use that will further enable this meta-analysis. Interpreters also engage in a "meta-frame" as they conduct their professional work, constantly recasting meaning within the other language. Both interpreters and speech-language pathologists, however, can fail to recognize each other's frames, and this can account for much of the "getting off on the wrong

foot" that can arise during interpreter-mediated interactions. Whereas speech-language pathologists seek to use interpreters' insights and judgments as a set of data (along with, for example, the judgments of patients, family members, and nursing staff), interpreters can feel as if they are being asked to step outside their role by providing such judgments. In the example provided, the matter being interpreted was concrete and related to the linguistic code, yet interpreters frequently are asked to comment on far more abstract and culturally laden matters. Friedland and Penn (2003), for example, discuss the complexities involved in an interpreter-mediated session involving what they describe as "cultural brokerage."

Isaac (2002a, 2002b) has stressed the important role of presession briefing in trying to set up a framework to negotiate such role alignments and shifts. Her work also demonstrates, however, the existence of a considerable power differential in the partnership, as revealed very tellingly in Example 5–2, drawn from her work. In this example of presession briefing, the speech-language pathologist dominates the interaction, explaining what will happen.

In this briefing, the speech-language pathologist provides only one explicit opportunity in turn-taking for the interpreter to seek clarification or to initiate a comment (turn 17: "Okay?"). Three points can be identified at which turn transitions might have occurred (turns 10, 12, 16), but in this session, the interpreter does not make use of these opportunities. In this situation, the two professionals have just completed another session, so perhaps prior negotiation has occurred. Another possibility is lack of experience: Less experienced interpreters may not know what

Example 5–2
Interpreter Presession Briefing

(*Key:* BC, backchannel; I, interpreter; P, patient;
S, speech-language pathologist.)

1	S:	This little boy is eight years and three months old . . .
BC	I:	Yes.
	S:	. . . and his name is . . . Ch . . . ? Is that how I say it?
2	I:	[*gives correct pronunciation*]
3	S:	I'm not sure who's going to be coming, but I'm assuming that mum [*unintelligible*] will be bringing him.
4	I:	They haven't arrived yet?
5	S:	Yeah, they're here already.
6	I:	Aha. They're here already.
7	S:	They've been here for a little while, so we'll just whiz through it. Um . . .
8	I:	Just quick.
9	S:	What I'm going to do . . . he's obviously older than the little one we did just then.
10	I:	Aha.
11	S:	So, I'm going to spend some time just chatting to mum, getting a bit of a history on how . . . ah . . . how his development's been going. Ah . . . um . . . I'm not sure of her English . . .
BC	I:	Mmhm.
	S:	. . . so, we'll see how we go . . . um . . . and probably do it through you anyway.
12	I:	Yes, okay.
13	S:	Um . . . then I'll spend some time with him, firstly assessing, like, his articulation . . .
BC	I:	Mmhm.
	S:	. . . because that was the main concern, but then I'll take a language sample.
14	I:	Mmhm.
15	S:	So, the language sample that I'm going to do is a storybook . . .
BC	I:	Mmhm.
	S:	. . . and I'm going to tell the story . . .
	I:	Mmhm.
	S:	. . . and I'm going to get him to retell it.
16	I:	Yes, okay.
17	S:	Okay?
18	I:	Aha.

Reproduced with permission of the author from: Isaac, K. (2002). *Breaking barriers, building bridges: Clinician-interpreter interaction in speech pathology practice.* Unpublished PhD thesis, University of Newcastle, Newcastle, Australia.

challenges lie ahead, or what needs to be negotiated. Certainly, from the example of the discourse that takes place during the session itself (i.e.,Example 5–1), it can be seen that perhaps the most important thing to be negotiated in the presession preparation between the two professionals is how online realignments, changes in footing, and shifts in frames or roles will be signaled and managed between the professionals.

Modeling Interprofessional Discourse

The issues highlighted in the interaction between interpreters and speech-language pathologists in the previous section apply equally to other interprofessional collaborations. Whenever different professionals work together, it is possible to see what Burger and Fillettaz (2002) call "an intersection of multiple social practices." The social practices of each professional grouping arise from the cultural discourse of that profession and shape what members from each grouping consider to be the appropriate contribution to the interaction, and also their "reading" of the activities of the other professional. Figure 5–1 provides a model of the multiple social practices involved in interprofessional discourse involving speech-language pathology, which involve the framing of the interprofessional interaction, and the relative footing in the interpersonal relationship between the interactants, and the assessment practices from which the findings in relation to the client/patient emerge.

The most common intersection between professions involves consul-

tation, and such consultation may take place with or without the presence of the person with the communication or swallowing disorder. The main issue affecting the discourse in such consultation is the cultural frame of reference that informs the understandings of each profession. Naturally, as discussed earlier, terminological confusions can arise here, but misunderstandings also can arise when cultural frames of reference differ. For example, as a speech-language pathologist seeks to consult with a teacher regarding the return to schooling of a child who has suffered traumatic brain injury, it is likely that the medical model, which attributes lack of attention and impulsivity to organic causes, is going to be discordant with the educational model, in which these difficulties are attributed to emotional or environmental causes (Chapman, Nasits, Challas, & Billinger, 1999). Beyond these more immediate sources of misunderstanding, it is important to consider the relative power and status for each of the professional frames involved. For example, the relative weight given to evidence-based paradigms is allied closely with differing levels of social status.

In addition to identifying each individual discipline and its contribution to the interaction, another important factor in interprofessional collaboration is the recognition of the consultation process as a unified discourse in itself. For example, the type of patient-related case conference common in rehabilitation settings creates what Maseide (2003) describes as a "socially distributed cognitive process" (pp. 372–373), as instantiated in the discourse of the group discussion. At the end of such a case conference, decisions about diag-

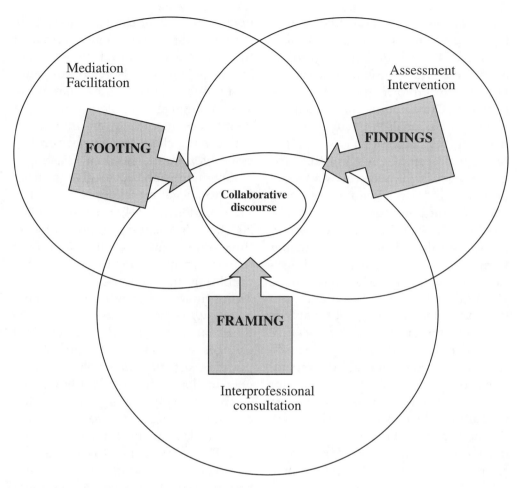

Figure 5–1. Multiple social practices.

nosis, prognosis, treatment goals, likely discharge destination, and so on have been made, but no one professional may be attributed with each decision or judgment. Maseide describes medical case conferences on patients with cancer and describes the interplay of explicit medical decision-making with the implicit interpersonal alignments required as moral problem-solving is negotiated in the team. Drawing on Goffman's work, Maseide draws attention to the way the medical frame creates the institutionalized footings of the members of the medical team (for example, hierarchies) but also how, in the moment-by-moment unfolding of the discourse, identities and alignments (footings) are created. As Maseide notes, "For this team to function a delicate balance is required between collegiality, equity, and recognition of special competence" (p. 399). In a study of interprofessional case conferences, Engestrom and colleagues identified three main ways in which such teams managed these tensions between professional and team goals and decision-making: articulation, cross-appropriation, and reconfiguration (Engestrom, Engestrom, & Keruso, 2003, p. 294). Articulation involved the explicit communication of professional knowledge or information to other professionals. Cross-appropriation occurred when professionals took up perspectives of other professionals. Reconfiguration was seen as emergent from the group discussions when new ways of thinking and decision-making arose from the interprofessional group discussion. The institutional discourse of the setting thus provides the broader frame for such locally negotiated decisions (Cook-Gumperz & Messerman, 1999), so that, in the rehabilitation setting example, "discharge" probably is the most important part of the case conference from the moment of admission, because the institutional imperative is reduced length of stay. Thus, for inpatient rehabilitation case conferences, the cultural ideology is primarily that of the medical model paradigm, in which discharge is the taken-for-granted assumed end point. The institutional imperatives preclude or marginalize other perspectives, with the issues of chronicity deferred to community settings. Therapy goals are reported by individual disciplines, but the shared goal in the discourse is that of discharge. The patient is absent from such case conferences and is represented through the discourse of the professionals. This representation, as in the matter of competence, for example, will have a major impact on the decisions that are made (Hall, Sarangi, & Slembrouck, 1999a, 1999b).

Figure 5–1 also illustrates the intersection of the issues surrounding the relative footing or alignment of the professionals working together to mediate or facilitate a client-clinician interaction. Although the most obvious example of this is the use of interpreters by speech-language pathologists in working with clients who speak another language, speech-language pathologists may find themselves mediating an interaction between the client and another professional, for example, when assisting a patient with aphasia to give instructions to a legal professional (Critchley, 1970; Enderby, 1994; Ferguson et al., 2004). Such discourse involves at least three interactants, so the alignment of participants shifts throughout the unfolding interaction—for example, as the clinician and other professional negotiate, as the clinician engages with the client, and as the other professional engages with the client. The relative power of each interactant will shape who gets the floor, when, and for how long.

The actual business of the session and the findings or outcomes of the session also are portrayed in Figure 5–1. This core business is the assessment or intervention processes and products of the main professional group involved and chiefly revolves around the clinician-client relationship. Although some of this core business continues in a unidisciplinary fashion, even when the other professional is absent, professionals may integrate interdisciplinary goals within their own sessions and interactions. For example, Lewis (2002) describes how generalization of a naming strategy for a person with aphasia was programmed into the occupational therapy sessions for the client.

At the central point of the interprofessional collaboration is an intersection of the purposes or agenda for the interaction of each participant (field) and the power and role relationships of the interactants (tenor); these factors will shape the way language is used in the interaction (mode). Figure 5–2 summarizes this intersection of purposes.

This intersection of collaborative practice can be viewed from the perspective of each participant. For the professionals involved, the purpose of the session probably will be the key factor deciding which professional takes the lead role in the interaction. This lead role is powerful, incorporating responsibility for involving establishing and maintaining rapport and directing the activities of the patient and the other professional(s). Within speech-language pathology sessions, the process is likely to be largely a metalinguistic endeavor (e.g., meta-textual, meta-pragmatic). For the other professional in any particular collaboration, the interpersonal roles are likely to proliferate and shift during the course of the interaction as the other professional mediates or facilitates or takes the

opportunity to carry out his or her own professional agenda. For the patient, some goals are essentially passive (to be assessed, treated), but goals also may be actively pursued, such as seeking to understand the problem or seeking to ensure that the professionals understand the degree of difficulties being experienced. The power of the patient in relation to the professionals is not straightforward, in that although the power to initiate and direct rests with the professionals, the patient holds considerable power to withhold, and in the three-way interaction, multiple opportunities emerge for the patient to align differentially with either of the professionals.

Expertise: Border Protection or Visa Application?

Such a model of interprofessional discourse provides the opportunity to look at some of the problems commonly

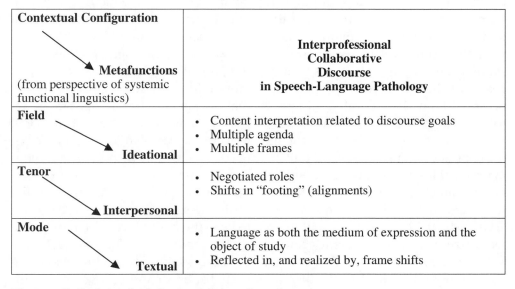

Figure 5–2. Interdisciplinary collaborative discourse.

encountered in interprofessional collaboration. In their presentation of an interdisciplinary approach to the management of feeding and swallowing disorders in children, Miller and colleagues discuss the difficulties raised when disciplines try to protect their professional territories (Miller et al., 2001). Territorial boundary protection is about power, and establishing which discipline is to be considered the most appropriate, the most competent, to carry out particular tasks. The role of power can be seen in the language used by these authors in their discussion: " . . . the occupational therapist and speech pathologist *may* assess a child's response to basic reinforcement strategies as traditionally would be assessed by the psychologist . . . however, *should defer* to the psychologist when the child and family require additional input and expertise with regard to establishing a formalized, behaviorally based feeding plan" [italics added] (Miller et al., p. 214). Not only do these authors explicitly describe the relationship between the professional groupings in terms of deference, but they note the implicit alignment of formalized plans with the profession to which greater status is attributed. This is not to suggest that different professions should or should not be allocated different roles in interprofessional collaboration, because clearly, role negotiation is at the heart of successful teamwork. Rather, in terms of the model presented in Figures 5–1 and 5–2, it can be predicted that turf wars will escalate when disputes arise in the field of discourse (failure to recognize or respect different agenda, failure to understand different uses of terminology), and it also can be suggested that the movement toward more transdisciplinary teamwork (as often seen in long established teams) is facilitated by multiparty sessions, wherein professionals have the opportunity to shift role relationships fluidly.

Published accounts of interprofessional practice tend to present idealized views of teamwork, in which better interpersonal communication is held to be the panacea for dysfunction in teams. In the real world, however, disputes that arise are not simply attributable to misunderstandings or personality or group dynamics. Professional perspectives do in fact differ with regard to frameworks for decision making, so situations arise in which individual professionals are doing battle on behalf of their institutional discourses. One of the paradoxes of expertise arises here, in that newly graduated speech-language pathologists can find themselves "instant experts" when they enter multidisciplinary teams, so that at a time when they are just beginning to integrate the theory and practice of the profession, they also are called on to justify, defend, and advocate for their professional perspective. Dimond (2006) provides a hypothetical example of such a dispute in the case of a patient with dysphagia for whom the recommendation is that the patient should receive nothing by mouth. In this situation, it was argued that the patient had the right to ignore professional advice, while at the same time the speech-language pathologist needed to remain with the recommendation based on the professional evidence base, and other members of the team (for example, nursing) also needed to keep their advice consistent with the recommendations. The nature of the better communication that handling such disputes requires involves a commitment to collaboration, rather than to individual disciplinary allegiances, and

Richards (2006) argues that small, committed, task-focused teams evidence substantial discoursal work in achieving consensual decision-making.

The development of training raises territory-related issues in interprofessional collaboration as assumptions are made regarding which profession is the "knower" and hence which profession is to train the other. This situation often is apparent in discussions of collaboration between teachers and speech-language pathologists; for example, in Mroz's description of training needs for early childhood teachers, she describes as a "joint working approach" a program in which teachers are trained and "closely supervised" and "overseen" by speech-language pathologists (Mroz, 2006, p. 168). The only point at which speech-language pathologists are seen as benefiting from this "collaboration" is in terms of obtaining assistance for dealing with the high caseload demand (p. 168). This profession-centric view perhaps reflects the nature of bureaucratic or institutionalized programs of training development and is in sharp contrast with more grounded collaborative work, such as that discussed by Tollerfield (2003). This investigator describes the collaborative work of speech language pathologists and teachers working in a special school environment, drawing on data from interviews, video recordings of classroom interaction, and diaries kept by the professionals. Findings from this qualitative research illustrate the full range of different types of interprofessional collaboration, from consultation (such as in relation to curriculum) to mediation (such as team teaching) to the routine teaching and therapy practices of each professional. In this collaborative project, power appeared to be equally distributed, with the description of the professional's respective approaches (field) reflecting this, for example, as evident in the following comment from a speech-language pathologist: "[teachers] are looking at things from a group point of view even if they're bringing it down to IEPs . . . we probably go from the individual upwards . . . [teachers] look at the group going down" (p. 72). The process of collaboration in mediating, facilitating each other's work is well accepted, as in Example 5–3.

In this example, from the work of Tollerfield (2003), the speech-language pathologist is facilitating the child's response (turns 9, 11) to the teacher's request (turns 1, 3, 5), but equally, the teacher's delivery of this part of the curriculum mediates the speech-language pathologist's goals for the child regarding phonological awareness. This very close collaboration facilitates the development of transdisciplinary skills, such that Tollerfield notes that both speech-language pathologists and teachers adopted each others forms of language use and communicative strategies over the period of the project.

The model presented in Figure 5–2 highlights that collaboration is most fully achieved through the intersection of both joint work with the client (mediation, facilitation) and joint work in consultation (e.g., planning, information sharing). As Nelson and Van Meter (2006) discuss in relation to work on literacy, the negotiation of roles in the joint work in the classroom is facilitated by understanding of each professional's theoretical perspectives. At the same time, these investigators note the fundamental importance of mutual respect and patience in the process of collaboration.

Example 5–3
Interprofessional Mediation in Education

(*Key:* J, Jayne [child client]; S, speech-language pathologist;
T, teacher ["Mrs. M"].)

1 T: We'll put the horse on the hat because . . . what does "horse"
       begin with, Jayne? . . . "horse" begins with . . .
2 J: [*no response*]
3 T: "Horse" [*heavily emphasized "h"*] . . . what does it begin with?
4 J: Horse.
5 T: It is a horse, but what can you hear at the beginning of the
       word? Listen . . . "horse" . . . [*heavily emphasized "h"*]
6 J: [*shaking head—no verbal response*]
7 S: Can I try something, Mrs. M?
8 T: Yes . . . yes . . . please do.
9 S: Jayne, this word says "horse" [*pointing to written word on display
       table*] . . . Here . . . it says "horse" . . . [*holding the word in front of
       Jayne*] Can you put your finger on the beginning of the word?
10 J: [*points to the "h"*]
11 S: Good . . . I'm going to cover the rest up. You have got your
       finger on the beginning of the word. What does it begin with?
12 J: "h."
13 T: Good girl.

From Tollerfield, I. (2003). The process of collaboration within a special school setting: An exploration of the ways in which skills and knowledge are shared and barriers are overcome when a teacher and speech and language therapist collaborate. *Child Language Teaching and Therapy, 19,* 67–84. (© Copyright Sage Publications, 2003, reproduced with permission Sage Publications Ltd)

Interprofessional Identity and Discourse

A major shift in the cultural conception of the nature of professional work has been occurring over the past two decades. As the work of service organizations becomes increasingly corporatized, the professional has changed from a notionally autonomous decision-maker, responsible for independent action within a highly specialized area, to that of an interdependent communicator responsible for collaboration within complex systems. As Engestrom and colleagues put it, "Medical work is no longer only about treating patients and finding cures. It is increasingly about reorganizing and reconceptualizing care across professional specialties and institutional boundaries" (Engestrom et al., 2003, p. 307). As services become increasingly integrated, professionals are expected to be increasingly multiskilled across a range of functions required by the workplace. Iedema and Scheeres (2003) used both ethnographic observations and interviews over a 2-year period to examine and contrast *total quality management* processes in a large factory setting and the *clinical pathway* processes in a large metropolitan hospital. The clinical pathway processes arose from government initiatives, and involved the development of interprofessional teams within hospital workplaces that sought to describe and construct an agreed-on statement as to the required steps and sequences for particular services provided to patients. In their research, Iedema and Scheeres found that these processes required the use of a "meta"-professional discourse: Each professional or worker needed to be able to talk about his or her work in ways that others would understand. Furthermore, the outcomes of such talk led to the construction of an identity in relation to the workplace, over that of the specific professional group. The researchers discuss the debate regarding whether, and to what extent, this cultural shift in workplaces is shifting the balance of power toward or away from workers. For example, the active participation in the construction and validation of the knowledge and practices within the workplace by workers would appear to shift power toward them. As suggested by these researchers, however, such processes as total quality management and clinical pathways may simply be more subtle means of manipulating and harnessing the energies of workers in the interests of the corporation.

Becoming an Expert in Interprofessional Discourse

The first major opportunity to learn about other professions involved in multidisciplinary care occurs in the initial professional preparation programs, but it appears that this opportunity is taken up to differing extents across the professional groups. Sullivan and Cleave (2003) surveyed 268 students from medicine, nursing, physiotherapy, and occupational therapy programs regarding their knowledge of speech-language pathology. Exposure to clinical experiences that involved a speech-language pathologist appeared to make the greatest impact on understanding the roles of the profession, with both occupational therapy and physiotherapy students knowing more and reporting more exposure than students from the other professions. Although the notion of multidisciplinary practice continues to be seen as valued, specific training in the skills needed to work well in teams continues to be far rarer than the educational efforts expended on the development of disciplinary expertise. Rodger and colleagues report on a training workshop developed with the aim of promoting interprofessional skills which was delivered to 81 graduate-entry allied health students (occupational therapy, speech-language pathology, physiotherapy, and audiology) through a 4-hour case-based workshop (Rodger, Mickan, Marinac, & Woodyatt, 2005). Before the workshop, less than one fifth of the students identified communication as important to teamwork, whereas after the workshop, one third of students reported that they had developed a better understanding of the communication skills required. Of interest, before the workshop, one quarter of the students considered that a common goal was important to teamwork, whereas after the workshop, this had dropped to less than one fifth. In relation to the model presented in Figure 5–2, this finding is of interest, because it raises the possibility that this interprofessional learning experience raised the students' awareness of the multiplicity of goals and agenda of diverse professionals and allowed for the development of the recognition of the legitimacy of other goals.

At times the educational goal of facilitating interdisciplinary skills veils what constitutes a form of "colonization" by other disciplines. Glista and Petersons (2003), for example, describe a gerontology curriculum designed for multiple disciplines (blind rehabilitation, community health, dental hygiene, dietetics, exercise science, occupational therapy, recreation, speech-language pathology, and audiology). In the implementation of this curriculum, each individual discipline learned about aspects of gerontology deemed to be important to allied health, and the aspects of interdisciplinary teamwork included in the curriculum were taught individually to each discipline.

Concluding Comments

In this chapter the discourse of interprofessional practice has been examined in terms of how disciplinary cultures influence the interaction of professionals as they consult and provide services. In many ways, the reality of "unidisciplinary practice" can be called into question—clients only rarely receive services from speech-language pathologists alone, and even in those instances, the speech-language pathologist is likely to draw on the institutional discourse of other disciplines (e.g., psychology, linguistics, education, medicine). The issue for practitioners becomes one of just how much collaboration will (or should) occur with other professionals. It is not always clear that the inclusion of increasing numbers of specialists enhances the quality of patient care, because both professionals and people with communication disorders (or their caregivers) make decisions about just who is involved and how. In particular, fragmentation can occur with increasing numbers of specialist professionals and threaten the provision of holistic patient care.

In summary, the important point here is that this interprofessional decision-making is mediated through discourse, most obviously in the face-to-face interactions that occur but also through the operation of the professional discourses informing practice, and through the operation of institutional discourses that direct and constrain service provision.

References

Burger, M., & Fillettaz, L. (2002). Media interviews: An intersection of multiple social practices. In C. N. Candlin (Ed.), *Research and practice in professional discourse* (pp. 567–588). Hong Kong: City University of Hong Kong Press.

Chapman, S. B., Nasits, J., Challas, J. D., & Billinger, A. P. (1999). Long-term recovery in paediatric head injury: Overcoming the hurdles. *Advances in Speech-Language Pathology, 1*(1), 19–30.

Cook-Gumperz, J., & Messerman, L. (1999). Local identities and institutional practices: Constructing the record of professional collaboration. In S. Sarangi & C. Roberts (Eds.), *Talk, work and institutional order: Discourse in medical, mediation and management settings* (pp. 145–181). Berlin: Mouton de Gruyter.

Critchley, M. (1970). *Aphasiology* (pp. 288–295). London: Edward Arnold.

Eadie, P. (2005). The case for public speech pathology terminology: Recognizing *Dianthus caryophyllus? Advances in Speech-Language Pathology, 7*(2), 91–93.

Enderby, P. (1994). The testamentary capacity of dysphasic patients. *Medico-Legal Journal, 62*(2), 70–80.

Engestrom, Y., Engestrom, R., & Keruso, H. (2003). The discursive construction of collaborative care. *Applied Linguistics, 24*(3), 286–315.

Ferguson, A., Candlin, C. N., Armstrong, E., Isaac, K., & Roger, P. (2005). *Speech pathologists and interpreters: Partners in action.* Paper presented at the 14th AILA World Congress of Applied Linguistics, Madison, WI, July 24–29.

Ferguson, A., Worrall, L., McPhee, J., Buskell, R., Armstrong, E., & Togher, L. (2004). *Autonomy in life decisions for people with aphasia: Issues for speech pathologists.* Paper presented at the 26th World Congress of the International Association of Logopedics & Phoniatrics, Brisbane, Australia, Aug. 29–Sept. 2.

Forrest, K. (2003). Diagnostic criteria of developmental apraxia of speech used by clinical speech-language pathologists. *American Journal of Speech-Language Pathology, 12*(3), 376–380.

Friedland, D., & Penn, C. (2003). Conversation analysis as a technique for exploring the dynamics of a mediated interview. *International Journal of Language & Communication Disorders, 38*(1), 95–111.

Glista, S., & Petersons, M. (2003). A model curriculum for interdisciplinary allied health gerontology education. *Gerontology & Geriatrics Education, 23*(4), 27–40.

Goffman, E. (1974). *Frame analysis: An essay on the organization of experience.* New York: Harper & Row.

Goffman, E. (1981). *Forms of talk.* Oxford: Basil Blackwell.

Hall, C., Sarangi, S., & Slembrouck, S. (1999a). The legitimation of the client and the profession: Identities and roles in social work discourse. In S. Sarangi & C. Roberts (Eds.), *Talk, work and institutional order: Discourse in medical, mediation and management settings* (pp. 293–322). Berlin: Mouton de Gruyter.

Hall, C., Sarangi, S., & Slembrouck, S. (1999b). Speech representation and the categorization of the client in social work discourse. *Text, 19*(4), 539–570.

Iedema, R., & Scheeres, H. (2003). From doing work to talking work: Renegotiating knowing, doing, and identity. *Applied Linguistics, 24*(3), 316–337.

Isaac, K. (2001). What about linguistic diversity? A different look at multicultural health care. *Communication Disorders Quarterly, 22*(2), 110–113.

Isaac, K., Roger, P., Candlin, C. N., Ferguson, A., & Armstrong, E. (2004). *Health care interpreters and speech pathologists: Exploring this professional partnership.* Paper presented at the 26th World Congress of the International Association of Logopedics and Phoniatrics, Brisbane, Australia, Aug. 29–Sept. 2.

Isaac, K. M. (2002a). *Breaking barriers, building bridges: Clinician-interpreter interaction in speech pathology practice.* Unpublished PhD thesis, University of Newcastle, Newcastle, Australia.

Isaac, K. M. (2002b). *Speech pathology in cultural and linguistic diversity.* London: Whurr.

Kamhi, A. G. (1998). Trying to make sense of developmental language disorders. *Language, Speech, and Hearing Services in Schools, 29*(1), 35–44.

Kertesz, A. (1982). *The Western Aphasia Battery*. New York: Grune & Stratton.

Kertesz, A. (2006). *Western Aphasia Battery —Revised*. San Antonio, TX: Harcourt Assessment.

Lewis, F. (2002). An interdisciplinary approach to naming ability. *Physical and Occupational Therapy in Geriatrics*, 20(3/4), 69–76.

Maseide, P. (2003). Medical talk and moral order: Social interaction and collaborative clinical work. *Text*, 23(3), 369–403.

Miller, C. K., Burklow, K. A., Santoro, K., Kirby, E., Mason, D., & Rudolph, C. D. (2001). An interdisciplinary team approach to the management of pediatric feeding and swallowing disorders. *Children's Health Care*, 30(3), 201–218.

Mroz, M. (2006). Providing training in speech and language for education professionals: Challenges, support and the view from the ground. *Child Language Teaching and Therapy*, 22(2), 155–176.

Nelson, N. W., & Van Meter, A. M. (2006). Partnerships for literacy in a writing lab approach. *Topics in Language Disorders*, 26(1), 55–69.

Plante, E. (1998). Criteria for SLI: The Stark and Tallal legacy and beyond. *Journal of Speech, Language, and Hearing Research*, 41, 951–957.

Richards, K. (2006). Staying onside: The negotiation of argument. In *Language and professional identity: Aspects of collaborative interaction* (pp. 55–91). Houndsmills, UK: Palgrave Macmillan.

Roberts, C., & Sarangi, S. (2003). Uptake of discourse research in interprofessional settings: Reporting from medical consultancy. *Applied Linguistics*, 24(3), 338–359.

Rodger, S., Mickan, S., Marinac, J., & Woodyatt, G. (2005). Enhancing teamwork among allied health students: Evaluation of an interprofessional workshop. *Journal of Allied Health*, 34(4), 230–235.

Roger, P. (2003). *Linguistic diversity and the assessment of aphasia*. Unpublished PhD thesis, University of Sydney, Sydney, Australia.

Schroeder, R. E., Fache, E. E., Morrison, M. P. H., Cavanaugh, C., West, M. P., & Fache, J. M. (1999). Improving communication among health professionals through education: A pilot study. *Journal of Health Administration Education*, 17(3), 175–198.

Seal, B. C. (2000). Working with educational interpreters. *Language, Speech, and Hearing Services in Schools*, 31(1), 15–25.

St. Louis, K. O., Raphael, L. J., Myers, F. L., & Bakker, K. (2003). Cluttering updated. *ASHA Leader*, November 18, 4–5, 20–22.

Sullivan, A., & Cleave, P. L. (2003). Knowledge of the roles of speech-language pathologists by students in other health care programs. *Journal of Speech-Language Pathology & Audiology*, 27(2), 98–107.

Tollerfield, I. (2003). The process of collaboration within a special school setting: An exploration of the ways in which skills and knowledge are shared and barriers are overcome when a teacher and speech and language therapist collaborate. *Child Language Teaching and Therapy*, 19, 67–84.

Ukrainetz, T. A., & Fresquez, E. F. (2003). "What *isn't* language?: A qualitative study of the role of the school speech-language pathologist. *Language, Speech, and Hearing Services in Schools*, 34(4), 284–298.

Walsh, R. (2005). Meaning and purpose: A conceptual model for speech pathology terminology. *Advances in Speech-Language Pathology*, 7(2), 65–76.

Webb, G. (2007). *Teachers' awareness of language impairment in primary-school-aged children*. Unpublished Masters of Arts (Honours) by Research, University of Newcastle, Newcastle, Australia.

6

Speech-Language Pathology Genres: Discourse Is Systematic

This chapter explores the types of discourse through which speech-language pathologists do their work. The focus here is on the written and spoken forms of discourse associated with speech-language pathology practice, as well as similarities to other types of discourse, such as interviewing and classroom discourse. Also, the ways in which the systematic nature of discourse allows experts to manipulate the resources of genres and registers are analyzed, leading to a consideration of the nature of therapy itself.

Culture and Types of Discourse

At some level, different sociocultural contexts commonly are observed to give rise to different types of discourse. Discourse analysts (particularly those working from the perspective of systemic functional linguistics), however, have attempted to describe the system-

atic ways in which language use changes in relation to context. The different types of discourse, described as *genres* (Fairclough, 2003), have particular "contextual configurations" (Hasan, 1985, 1994) comprising *field* (what is going on in the interaction), *tenor* (the interpersonal role relationships between the interactants), and *mode* (how language is being used in the interaction). So, for example, progress notes in the medical record of a person with a communication disorder have the purpose of documenting the clinician's actions in relation to the patient, and the patient's communication status at that time (i.e., field) and are written by the clinician and directed to other professionals in their clinical roles, as well as for a potential legal audience (i.e., tenor); the record also is written for delayed reading by others unseen by the writer (i.e., mode). The contextual configuration of this genre is markedly different from that of the assessment session, the purpose of which is to determine the nature and severity of the communication difficulties (field), involving the interactants in their role relationship of clinician and patient (tenor), and mediated through both speaking and writing in face-to-face immediate contact (mode). These different contextual configurations of different types of discourse are systematically related to the linguistic resources used by the interactants in each genre. This system of relationships is one that is seen as probabilistic rather than deterministic in nature—in other words, certain configurations of contextual features are highly likely to involve, but do not inevitably involve, certain constellations of linguistic choices.

The structure of genres is described in terms of *elements* (which may be obligatory or optional for the identity of the genre) and *sequences of elements* (which may be in fixed order or unordered or occur recursively) (Hasan, 1985; Martin, 1997). The notion of the genre of texts is akin to the notion of the mental representation of schema or scripts, and it is through experience with genres in the discourse of daily life that these mental representations develop (Labov & Waletzky, 1967; Rumelhart, 1975), that is, through social contexts. Whereas the term *genre* is used to describe the structure of text types, the term *register* describes how language is used across the elements of the genre; that is, register describes the particular set of linguistic choices that interactants make within a genre. As Christie expresses this relationship: "A genre is a staged, purposive activity in which certain significant goals are achieved: its various stages or elements of structure are built through changing sets of register choices . . . " (Christie, 1997, p. 158).

So, within the genre of progress notes, the clinician will refer to the patient in the third person and is likely to nominalize events (for example, "the assessment showed" versus "I assessed"), and no opportunity exists for the patient to make a contribution to the exchange of information, but in the assessment session, the clinician will refer to the patient in the second person and is likely to actively describe processes, and opportunity is present for the patient to contribute to the exchange. Shifts in register provide a way in which interactants can manipulate the resources available within the genre, and indeed change the genre, so it can be seen that the system of discourse provides for a two-way relationship between the context of situation and the use of language. For example, a clinician may subvert the genre of progress notes in order to make a covert political statement in a situation in which perhaps time allotted for assessment of the patient was inadequate because of funding constraints.

This chapter considers some of the most common genres in speech-language pathology in both written and spoken discourse, as well as some of the aspects of register that illuminate the wider sociocultural context of professional practice.

Written Genres in Speech-Language Pathology

One of the first genres encountered in students beginning their professional education in speech-language pathology is not specific to the discipline, because novice students typically first are engaged with writing for academic purposes. Within the academic genres, Veel discusses how students in secondary education move to increasing expertise through working through a hierarchy of cognitive demand, from sequential recounts of information or observations through causal, then factorial, and finally theoretical explanations (Veel, 1997). By the time of entry into tertiary education, Woodward-Kron's analysis of academic writing suggests that students make use of embedded genres to learn and display learning—so, for example, in essentially expository pieces of written discourse, students use linking paragraphs to provide evaluative comment (Woodward-Kron, 2005). These written texts are argued by Woodward-Kron to differ substantially from the actual discourses of the discipline (Woodward-Kron, 2002). She proposes that as novices move toward expert status, a movement occurs from pedagogical discourse to the disciplinary discourse. So, for example, textbooks present knowledge as static bodies of known information, whereas the discourse of the discipline recognizes that knowledge is constructed, dynamic, and unknown. She suggests that the way students make this transition is through the critical analysis that takes place through the comparison and contrasting of multiple texts. These multiple texts for students learning to be speech-language pathologists are drawn from both the academic and workplace environment; that is, it is not only the written texts of research in the discipline and the spoken discourse of lectures but also the experience of

observing and participating in assessment and treatment of people with communication disorders that shapes this evolution toward expertise in the disciplinary discourse.

In the academic environment, the learner's experience is staged across increasing levels of cognitive demand. In the workplace, however, Beaufort's ethnographic research suggests that novices are assigned writing tasks in terms of least importance to the institution's goals, working their way up to tasks of greater importance to the institution (Beaufort, 2000). So, for example, internal memos may be undertaken by novices, but submissions for funding or positions would be undertaken by senior experts. Just as novice students who are involved in writing progress notes, for example, will be provided with modeling, scaffolding, and feedback by their educator, so too is it likely that the less experienced clinician will be mentored or directly supervised (perhaps through coauthoring) for written tasks of more importance to the institution. The development of writing in terms of acquisition of written genres in the academic and workplace environments continues with the development of expertise (and, as with any other expertise development, requires specific attention, rather than simply accumulating experience). For example, the genre of the written thesis (Kwan, 2006) is very distinct from clinical reporting, and the genre of the written journal article is very different from the conventions associated with written submissions for funding in the workplace. The mastery of these genres reflects the expertise of the writer and also brings with it greater opportunities for the exertion of power within both the academic and workplace environments.

The development of writing skills for both academic and workplace environments means developing an understanding of the structural requirements of the genre, and of the linguistic resources within the registers considered appropriate to the genre. The acquisition of expertise requires the development of a kind of critical literacy, such that the writer can recognize that although opinions are in fact expressed across the genres of the personal letter, the essay, and scientific writing (including the clinical report), the way language is used to express opinion differs in each genre (Hood, 2005; Hyland, 2005). Some groups of students are especially disadvantaged in relation to use of the types of genre associated with the writing demands of the academic and workplace environments, as a result of cultural unfamiliarity, the need for writers to use their second language, or socioeconomically disadvantaged status. Hood (2005) argues that simply identifying ways to make such writers more aware of the linguistic requirements of the task is not enough, suggesting that the barrier of prescribed writing genres effectively silences the cultural voice of students from different backgrounds, either through their failure to master the genre—and so failing and leaving the pathway to professional work—or through successfully mastering the genre, so that their voices, as Fairclough suggests, merge with the dominant ideology and differences cease to be expressed (Fairclough, 1989).

The critical literacy movement argues that the way through this dilemma is to raise students' awareness of different discourses and their sociocultural and sociopolitical ideologies and consequences (Fernsten, 2005). This need for the development of critical literacy applies to all students, and indeed all experts, because the status quo for writing in the workplace in the practice of speech-language pathology is arguably problematic (Duchan, 1999), with clinical reports in particular failing to communicate effectively with the intended audiences, instead reflecting professional ideological assumptions regarding the competence of clients and the role of experts (see Chapter 2). A first step toward this kind of cultural literacy is the explicit recognition of different genres as culturally embedded, rather than regarding writing as being more or less "correct." Higgs and colleagues provide an example of guidance to students developing academic writing skills that explicitly identifies the role of cultural conventions (Higgs, McAllister, & Rosenthal, 2005), as well as practical guidance for the development of written expertise.

Spoken Genres in Speech-Language Pathology

One-to-One Interaction

The most readily identified spoken genres in speech-language pathology are those of assessment and treatment sessions, and in essentials, these session genres relate to other more widely recognized social genres. As illustrated in Figure 6–1, the assessment session reflects the genre of the interview, and

Contextual aspect of discourse	Interview (medical history, examination)	Speech-language pathology assessment session	Therapeutic interview (counseling)	Lesson (classroom discourse)	Speech-language pathology treatment session
Field	Investigation of presenting problem	Investigation of presenting problem	Promotion of change in attitudes (affect)	Promotion of change in knowledge, skills, or attitudes	Promotion of change in knowledge, skills, or attitudes
Tenor	Physician-patient Power asymmetry	Clinician-client Power asymmetry	Clinician-client Power asymmetry	Teacher-student(s) Power asymmetry	Therapist-client(s) Power asymmetry
Mode	Spoken, written Language as action	Spoken, written Language as action	Spoken, written Language as action	Spoken, written Language as action	Spoken, written Language as action

Figure 6–1. Contextual configuration of assessment and treatment sessions.

in particular the medical interview and examination. The treatment session reflects the genre of the lesson, in particular classroom discourse. The cross-disciplinary context of therapy, however, often means that elements of classroom discourse are evident within speech-language pathology assessment, and that elements of the medical interview are evident within speech-language pathology treatment. Similarly, crossover between genres is evident in the therapeutic counseling interview, because this genre shares features with both the interview and lesson genres, and the counseling aspect of speech-language treatment shares many features with the therapeutic interview.

Previous research on the nature of assessment and treatment genres in speech-language pathology has identified the temporal ordering of broad stages within the session. For the *assessment* session, Ferguson and Elliot (2001) describe these stages as greeting, rap-

port building, procedural orientation, case history, observation and testing, provision diagnosis and description, plan, and leave-taking. Research into the related genre of the medical interview has focused on the case history stage in particular, noting the asymmetries in the interaction and the constraints on clients' contributions (Buchwald et al., 1993; Hein & Wodak, 1987; West, 1984). In speech-language pathology, similar asymmetries have been reported within assessment sessions, particularly when sessions involve persons from culturally different backgrounds (Hand, 2001, 2003, 2006).

For the *treatment* session, Horton (2006) describes stages within the session as the "settling down period," "opening up the business," "doing therapy tasks," and the "closing down period." Research into the related genre of classroom discourse has focused on moments involving direct instruction, influenced strongly by models of such teaching in terms of initiation-response-feedback[1] cycles (Sinclair & Coulthard, 1975). In speech-language pathology, a similar focus is evident, making use of the same model (Horton & Byng, 2000). The initiation-response-feedback cycle has considerable face-validity in the field, given the strong behaviorist tradition that underpins (implicitly or explicitly) speech-language intervention, and previous analytical tools to describe sessions have been largely behavioral in focus (Boone & Prescott, 1972; Brookshire, 1976). Lewis and Hand (1998) critique the applicability of this type of model, arguing that the initiation-response-feedback cycle does not capture much of what is going on in child language therapy, in view of therapy rationales related to sociocognitive mediation of language development, rather than behavioral modification.

An alternative approach to the description of assessment and treatment is to consider how the resources of the genres and their associated registers are used by the interactants. So, for example, research looking at a series of single case descriptions found that the proportion of the session devoted to rapport building increased with increased expertise of novice students, experienced students, and expert speech-language pathologists in the assessment and treatment of stuttering and aphasia (Ferguson, 1998; Ferguson & Elliot, 2001). This finding is consistent with Laufer and Glick's work on everyday experts, in which the experts did more rapport building with cus-

tomers—for example, "sizing up" the person, engaging in dialogic negotiation, or seeking longer-term relationship building (Laufer & Glick, 1996). Thus, the element of rapport building is structurally an "option" in the generic structure of sessions but an important one that experts exploit to achieve their goals.

Another important structural element involves the stage of therapy described by Ferguson (1998) and Ferguson and Elliott (2001) as "procedural orientation" and by Horton (2006) as "task introduction." Horton suggests that this introduction is where the linguistic or cognitive demands of the task are set out for the patient. In research into the structure of stuttering assessment and treatment sessions involving two novice students, an experienced student, and an expert speech-language pathologist, procedural orientation was evident in all assessment sessions but surprisingly did not occur in stuttering treatment sessions (Ferguson, 1998). Possibly, considerable knowledge was shared between clinician and client about the nature of therapy tasks in the behavioral stuttering management programs that were being conducted in these sessions; alternatively, it could be asked whether at that stage of the clinician-client relationship, control had been fully taken or handed over, with the patient playing a passive role in the therapeutic process. In the investigation of aphasia treatment sessions, however, procedural orientation was evident in all sessions, taking up 2.6% of the novice student's moves,

---

[1]Broadly synonymous versions of these terms include *elicitation–response–follow-up* and *request–response–evaluation*. In this book, the term *initiation-response-feedback* is used as an equivalent set.

10.8% of the experienced student's moves, and 1.9% of the expert speech-language pathologist's moves (Ferguson & Elliot, 2001). The influence of increasing levels of expertise is evident from the examination of examples of these clinicians' procedural orientations in working with people with severe aphasia who had significantly restricted verbal expression with relatively spared auditory comprehension; see Examples 6–1, 6–2, and 6–3.

In Example 6–1, the novice student is seen to adopt a modalized register, such that instructions are hedged—for example, in turn 1, "I've *just* got. . . ." The novice student does explicitly direct the patient in turn 1, "*you* have to . . . ," but switches to the inclusive "we" by turn 3: "*we*'re just going to. . . . " In engaging with the issue of the com-plexity of the task, the novice clinician switches to a depersonalized form in turn 3: "*they*'re going to get harder"—perhaps as a strategy to minimize the face-threat associated with assumption of difficulty. The novice student's attempt at humor in turn 7, "you're armed, you're ready . . . ," possibly is another strategy to try to manage the positioning of clinician and patient, because this utterance aligns the patient with (or against) the task, rather than with the clinician as the source of learning (or potential difficulty). Noticeably absent from the novice student's procedural orientation is any rationale for the activity: No explanation is provided to the patient of why doing the activity will be of benefit.

In Example 6–2, the experienced student uses a heavily modalized register

---

Example 6–1
Novice Student Procedural Orientation

(*Key:* P, patient; S, student)

(This was the first and only procedural orientation element in this session, occurring after an initial period of rapport building. The patient had severe aphasia restricting verbal expression, with relatively spared auditory comprehension.)

1   S: All right, what we're going to do today is . . . I've just got some tasks that just involve you writing and filling in the gap of the sentence, okay? So like: "drive the . . . " and you have to fill in the word for me, okay? So I've put all the words at the top here.

2   P: I saw that.

3   S: And they're going to get harder, like next time I don't give you any clues . . . and we're just going to see how we go.

4   P: Mm.

5   S: Okay? This is sort of similar to what we were doing last week.

6   P: Yep.

7   S: All right. Okay, you're armed, you're ready . . . okay.

> ## Example 6–2
> ## Experienced Student Procedural Orientation
>
> (*Key:* P, patient; S, student; < >, overlapping speech; XXX, unintelligible.)
>
> (This was the first procedural orientation element in this session and the first part of the recorded interaction. The patient had severe aphasia restricting verbal expression, with relatively spared auditory comprehension.)
>
> 1 S: Yeah, yep. I see. Well, I didn't bring any news today—I thought we might leave that till next week . . . I might bring you some . . . some radio broadcasts . . . for next week. I thought I'd give that a break since we did some last week. So we'll do something a bit different.
>
> 2 P: Okay, "S" [*name of student*].
>
> 3 S: Is that okay? Now . . . I've brought you some timetables to have a look at, but I thought what I might start with today is going back over . . . um . . . our "wh-" questions, if that's <all right.>
>
> 4 P: <XXX.>
>
> 5 S: Yep. Who, where, when, what, why—all those sort of things . . . so we'll do some more from that. It's just sort of following on from when we were doing . . . um . . . the headlines on the articles and that sort of thing? Yeah? So that's good just to get you cueing in to . . . um . . . the important information. Okay? So what I'm going to do is just ask—just read a sentence to you and ask you "who" or "what" or some questions like <that.>
>
> 6 P: <Yes.>
>
> 7 S: Is that okay?
>
> 8 P: Yes.
>
> 9 S: All right. So they're pretty . . . yeah . . . we've been doing some maybe three- or four-sentence packages. These ones are just one sentence so you'll probably find them pretty easy, but that's okay, isn't it? [*Laughs.*]

throughout (for example, turn 1, "I *thought* we *might* . . . "), with constant checks with the patient (for example, " . . . if that's all right" in turn 3 and "Is that okay?" in turn 7). This checking also was seen in the novice student's procedural orientation and may represent an attempt to bring the patient into the process of negotiating the task.

Again, the inclusive "we" is used—for example in turn 1, "*we* did . . . *we*'ll do . . . "—and at no point is the explanation framed directly with reference to what "you," the patient, is being asked to do. Instead, the experienced student depersonalizes the instruction aspect of the procedural orientation through the use of complex clausal constructions that turn the focus from the patient back to the clinician's activity, for example, in turn 3, "I've brought *you* some timetables *to have a look* at . . . ," and turn 5, "what I'm going to do is just ask—just read a sentence *to you* and *ask you* who or what or some questions like that." Unlike the novice student, the experienced student directly addresses the issue of the complexity of the task in turn 9: " . . . you'll probably find them pretty easy . . . "; the hesitancy and reformulations evident in this turn, however, suggest that this issue is problematic for the student. The experienced student does attempt the inclusion of the rationale for the task in turn 5: " . . . to get you cueing in to . . . um . . . the important information."

In Example 6–3, the expert speech-language pathologist addresses the same issues attempted by the students, but more efficiently. She too hedges, for example, in turn 5, "we *might just* . . . ," but this is not a feature of the register she is using. She makes use of the inclusive "we" pervasively throughout the procedural orientation—for example, in turn 1, "*we*'ve been practicing your gestures. . . . " The direct use of *you* also arises in relation to the focus of the task in turn 1, " . . . practicing *your* gestures," and in the explanation of the rationale of the task, in turn 3, " . . . if *you* can use them, as—well, as trying to talk that will help get *your* message across." She also engages with task complexity, but only indirectly, through

---

Example 6–3
Expert Procedural Orientation

(*Key:* C, clinician; P, patient; < >, overlapping speech.)

(This was the first procedural orientation element in this session, occurring after a period of rapport building. The patient had severe aphasia and severe apraxia of speech restricting verbal expression, with relatively spared auditory comprehension.)

1	C:	All right. So one of the things we've been practicing, okay . . . is your gestures. So . . . using your hands more to show what's <happening.>
2	P:	<Yeah.>
3	C:	To help get your message across . . . okay. So we've been practising some of these. Okay . . . and I think if you can use them, as . . . well as trying to talk, that will help get your message across.
4	P:	Yeah.
5	C:	All right—okay. So we might just run through them first, because it's a couple of days since we've done them.
6	P:	Mm.
7	C:	We'll just run through them so you remember what they <are.>
8	P:	<Mm.>

indicating the need for a review of previous practice (in turns 5 and 7).

The greater efficiency of the expert speech-language pathologist seen in the register used in procedural orientation also was seen in use of all of the structural resources of the session genre. As Horton (2006) discusses, each element within the session is not a separate module but rather sets up or follows through aspects of the learning interaction that arise within other elements. Procedural orientation is a very visible instance of mediation of the action of therapy, and how it is integrated within the session reflects the way in which the therapeutic process is mediated. The novice student from the previously discussed data engaged in procedural orientation only once and at the start of the session, whereas the experienced student recursively engaged in procedural orientation before each therapy activity, the organization of which can be expressed as ⌐(PO ^ TA) (where PO is procedural orientation and TA is therapy activity). For the expert, however, procedural orientation was both recursive and embedded within a more complex recursive set that included both review of progress (REV) and planning for the future (P), which can be expressed as ⌐{PO ^ ⌐(TA ^ REV) ^ P}.

Across all data researched to date regarding procedural orientation is the striking absence of collaborative involvement of the patient. Procedural orientation was all about what the clinician was "doing to" the patient, even though, because these patients retained reasonably adequate auditory comprehension, negotiation would be possible about the purpose of the task and the rationale for why doing the task would be of benefit. As Horton has stated with reference to his data from 15 aphasia therapy sessions: "Therapists make efforts to provide explanations about tasks, but it is hard to see from these data how anyone other than a professional insider could really understand the reasoning behind the suggested relative difficulty of tasks" (Horton, 2006, p. 548). Without such understanding of specific tasks, clients are prevented from understanding what it is they are trying to do in terms of the clinician-directed goals for therapy. Without negotiation toward a shared understanding of the point of therapy, then the goals of clients in therapy may never be met (Worrall et al., 2006). Explanation in the absence of client collaboration raises important questions about the role of providing orientation to tasks. As Horton has observed, "Therapists may seek to maintain their expert status by not displaying evidence of their own thinking or reasoning processing" (Horton, p. 560). In other words, procedural orientation serves to instantiate the power of the therapist and sets up the social positioning of the person with a communication disorder as "patient" or "client" through this form of regulative discourse.

The element within the genre of the therapy session to which the client can be seen to make the largest contribution as an equal partner occurs in the opening stages, involving casual conversation. As previously mentioned, the data on novice to expert sessions in aphasia and stuttering (Ferguson, 1998; Ferguson & Elliot, 2001) revealed an increasing proportion of moves involving rapport building associated with increasing experience. In view of the interrelationship between the work done within each element and that occurring in other elements, it is suggested that "chat" is used by the expert to mediate therapeutic action. A parallel with these observations has been recognized within speech-language pathology sessions and in the related classroom genres (Christie, 1997). Christie notes the interplay of regulative discourse and instructional discourse in "morning news," a particular genre associated with the classroom and in relation to what she refers to as other classroom learning activities running across a series of lessons. She notes that in morning news, the regulative register is separate from the instructional register, in that the teacher sets up the control and rules of the interaction and closes the interaction, but the topic content is essentially open to the students' choices. In the classroom-themed learning activities, however, the regulative and instructional registers are integrated, such that the teacher is controlling both the "how" and the "what" of the discourse. This example relates closely to the opening chat between clinician and client, in which, as Horton (2006) notes, the clinician sets up the power relationship of control, although the client has choices regarding what is contributed. This regulative register then is integrated with the instructional register in what Horton describes as "doing therapy." Christie suggests that this integration of regulative and instructional registers is the mechanism by which the teacher can be seen as an agent of "symbolic control" (p. 157)—that is, the teacher's discourse is the means by which the social positioning of the child as learner is instantiated. In a similar way, the therapist's discourse can be seen as the means by which the

social positioning of the child or adult with communication disorder is created. In the foregoing examples and in Horton's data, this social positioning is as passive recipient of therapy, rather than director or collaborator.

Thus far, these considerations regarding speech-language pathology genres have focused on one-to-one interaction. Do the issues with regard to power in particular also apply in group interactions involving people with communication disorders?

Group Interaction

Group interactions in speech-language pathology generally are associated with therapy, and tend to fall within two broad types: those in which the goal is to facilitate change in specific communicative behaviors and those in which the goal is to facilitate psychosocial improvements related to quality of life for persons with communication disorders. Group therapy targeting specific communicative behaviors tends to be very similar to individual therapy in that the therapist controls the session throughout, orchestrating communication between group participants for the purposes of providing practice in particular activities. In an analysis of this type of group interaction, Kovarsky and colleagues (1999) demonstrated that such interaction can result in the construction of incompetence, rather than development toward competence, through the requirement that contributions by group members be "correct" in relation to eliciting constraints of the therapist, rather than the communicative purposes of such contributions being locally negotiated by the group participants.

Even when clinicians attempt to facilitate the second type of group therapy, aiming for psychosocial support, patterns of interaction associated with behavioral therapy cross into the realm of psychosocial therapy. Markova (1991) describes the analysis of group sessions with adults with learning disability that were planned to be conversational in nature, with the aim of providing opportunities for these adults to have communicative opportunities for initiation outside those typically experienced. Markova describes typical therapy interchanges as adequately captured by Sinclair and Coulthard's "initiation-response" model (Sinclair & Coulthard, 1975) but notes that in conversation, each contribution has a "Janus-like" quality, such that each response becomes the initiation of subsequent contributions, and so on (Markova, 1991). In the group sessions that had aimed to provide for conversational opportunities, it was found that the clinicians continued to adopt the isolated initiation-response sequence, repeatedly taking the initiation move and directing clients within the group for the response. When group members did respond to responses, that is, initiate moves, these moves were not pursued by the clinicians, and it was only when the clinician was absent or inattentive that the group members engaged in truly conversational interchanges. Conversational exchange within group therapy aiming for social support is the vehicle for achieving the aims of such groups to facilitate the growth and adaptation of social identity for group members (Shadden & Agan, 2004), and if groups with those aims are structured and facilitated in ways more associated with behavioral

therapy, then the group process will construct the identity of "passive patient," rather than "social participant." That said, it can be challenging for the clinician to develop the skills required to facilitate this participation, because the institutional role and inherent power asymmetry of communicative competence involved in such an "inter-ability" encounter (Fox & Giles, 1996; Watson & Gallois, 2002) will constantly work to subvert the achievement of the goal of equal participation, as illustrated in Example 6–4.

Example 6–4 is taken from a audio/video recording of an interaction between group members in an aphasia group therapy program using a psychosocial conversational framework which has been demonstrated to improve overall communicative effectiveness, reported self-esteem, and quality of life (Alston, Sherratt, Ferguson, & Vajak, 2006). Twelve participants were engaged in this interaction, six of whom contributed verbally at the moment captured in this example—all seated around a table, with two video cameras at opposite corners used to record the interaction. Of the silent participants, two were speech-language pathology students, and four were persons with aphasia. Of the participants who contributed verbally, two were speech-language pathologists (S1, S2) and four were persons with mild-moderate aphasia (P1, P2, and P4 had fluent aphasia; P3 had nonfluent aphasia). In this example, the S1 clinician tends to direct her queries to the group in general, rather than eliciting responses from particular group members (for example, in turn 1, "Anyone going to . . . ?"), and both clinicians (S1 and S2) respond to the responses of each other

Example 6–4
Group Interaction

(*Key*: C1, clinician 1; C2, clinician 2; P1, P2, P3, P4, patients 1 to 4;
< >, overlapping speech.)

(This exchange occurred about 9 minutes into the group session, during discussion of plans for a night out. The patients all had mild-moderate aphasia. Four other patients and two speech-language pathology students also were engaging nonverbally in this interaction (refer to seating layout below).

1   C1:   Okay, good-oh—all organized. It'll be a good night. [*P2 laughs.*]
          Anyone going to do some ballroom dancing while you're there?
2   P1:   No [*laughingly*].
3   C2:   [*To P1*] Apparently they do ballroom <dancing there.>
4   P1:   [*To C2*] <Yeah, I used to> do ballroom dancing there.
5   C2:   [*To P1*] Really.
6   C1:   [*To P1*] Did you?
7   C1:   "P2" and "wife"—you might get up and have a dance?
8   P2:   Oh yes.
9   P3:   [*To P4*] You?
10 P4:   Eh? [*laughingly*].
11 P3:   You, "P4"—get up and dance?
12 P4:   Can't understand [*laughingly*]. [*General laughter from group.*]
13 C1:   Any excuse, any excuse [*laughingly*].

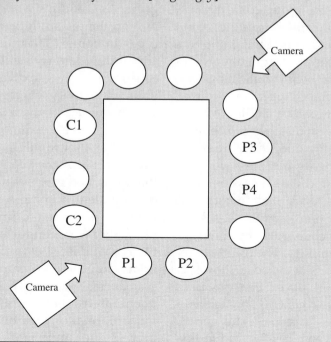

and group members (thereby transforming group member responses to initiations), for example, in turn 6, "Did you?" The initiation by P3 in turn 9 ("You?") directed toward P4 opens up an exchange that involves all 12 group members. Here, P4 uses the opportunity to direct his response back to the group as a whole, rather than solely to P3, for humorous purposes as he invokes his identity as someone with aphasia to provide a mock excuse for not answering the question about whether he would or would not be dancing at the next group outing (turn 12)— "Can't understand." The clinician (S1) underscores his humorous intent in turn 13 ("any excuse"), possibly for the benefit of group members with reduced comprehension. Thus, this example illustrates some of the important differences between behaviorally versus socially targeted therapies, as well as illustrating some of the identity work that emerges through the discourse within the group context.

Of course, the differences drawn out here between individual and group contexts are dissociable from the genres associated with behavioral change versus psychosocial change. For example, group sessions can be similar to classroom discourse in that they can be structured so that the one leader treats the many participants as if they were one person. Also, individual sessions with a counseling focus may incorporate features of the unfolding {I→RI→R . . . } sequence which is seen in conversational group settings. The feature of the interactions considered so far, however, is that they all have been described within a confined generic structure associated with the "session." This generic concept is challenged in the next section.

Social Construction of Therapy

The social identity of the therapist is constructed through the institutional discourse of the community, such as through recognition of qualifications and experience, but this social identity is also constructed locally through the interaction with people with communication disorders in their role as client. Construction of the client identity is achieved through the discourse of the "session" (Hagstrom & Wertsch, 2004). But if a person who is a speech-language pathologist is interacting with a person who has a communication disorder outside the "session" construct, to what extent is the former person's social identity still that of a therapist, and how are therapeutic interactions mediated outside the social construction of a session? To explore this issue, it is useful to return to the notion of genre: In Bakhtin's work, spoken and written genres are integral to activity types in context (Bakhtin, 1986) and, although "relatively stable" (p. 60) and constrained by context, reflect the individual creativity of the participants who make use of the resources of the genre to make meaning. In practical terms, this contextual fluidity of genres can be seen in the report of research that examined entire morning sessions of outpatient hospital services (rather than just individual case history interviews that were conducted during that time) (Wodak, 1996). This research underscored the disempowerment of patients in this setting, in the face of frequent interruptions and failure to provide information regarding purpose or processes for investigative procedures, with miscommunication associated with lack of shared understanding regarding the type of discourse expected and occurring across both staff and patients. As genres "slip," interactants can find themselves uncertain regarding their communicative role.

In Leahy's analysis of a stuttering therapy session, she notes that the speech-language pathologist appeared to be trying to construct a conversational exchange on two occasions during the session in order to provide opportunities for the client to maintain fluency-enhancing strategies in this genre, but on the first attempt ran into difficulty through providing corrective feedback and on the second attempt returned to more classical therapy after 8 turns, possibly because of apparent hesitancy demonstrated by the client. At a theoretical level, the question is about what it is that defines a particular genre (Grossen & Orvig, 1998), but in clinical practice, the question is the extent to which the interaction is "therapeutic" when the hallmark features of the therapy genre are not evident.

These questions arise in the everyday work of speech-language pathologists. For example, administrators query not so much the purpose of group therapy for aphasia or support programs for parents of children with disability, but whether it takes a speech-language pathologist's involvement for these groups to achieve their ends. These questions also arise for clinicians who over time develop personal relationships with children or adults formerly or currently in therapy—when are they friends, and when are they therapists? These questions arise, too, in the everyday discussions with speech-language pathology students as they seek out

increased hours of experience in sessions while devaluing or indeed failing to recognize the therapeutic goals and activities of home visits, functional real-life problem-solving, and time spent "just talking" in groups with people with communication disorders and with other people involved in their lives. When Byng and Black (1995) asked, "What makes a therapy?" the answer came back to the description of aspects of the therapeutic environment (e.g., stimuli, cues, contingencies), and when Ferguson (1999) tackled the same issue, the answer came down to the rationale resting on the likelihood of changing something that someone else does. Both answers fail to recognize therapy as socially mediated, whether by social action or through discourse. The recognition of the importance of mediation leads to the recognition that it is the two-way nature of the relationship between the person-as-therapist and the person-as-client that constitutes therapy—it is the "other" focus of both interactants than defines the moment as therapy. Grossman and Orvig (1998) suggest that rather than looking to structural linguistic features to identify and describe clinical genres, it is the intersubjectivity involved that identifies the clinical genres—that is, the joint conception of purpose, the process of the joint construction of an understanding of the problem, and shared work in the remediation of the problem. In this more fluid conception of genre, it becomes apparent that the often observed asymmetry of clinical interactions is not an inevitable feature of the discourse and yet also is an available resource for both clinicians and clients to exploit, for example, in providing reassurance or in displaying that they are actively listening (ten Have, 1991). Examination of the discourse in interactions between therapists and clients outside the session will evidence the traces of therapeutic discourse, not so much embedded as integrated within the exchange. So, for example, the initiation-response-feedback cycle associated with therapy sessions is transposed within conversation to, say, the therapist's use of a slower rate of speech accompanied by gesture in the conversational move equivalent to the initiation component, and the use of feedback that is less explicit than in the context of session (because "good" is an obviously inappropriate follow-up move in conversation) but more explicit than is typically used in conversation (such as "I understood that" instead of using backchanneling). Such therapeutic discourse would show active engagement of the client in explicit comment and contribution to the development of understanding, skill, or feelings about communication. That is, therapeutic discourse is not covert; it is explicitly available for comment and negotiation by both interactants—it is not only socially constructed but also socially recognizable to the interactants. Even in therapies that diverge considerably from initiation-response-feedback models, such as narrative or discourse therapies, it can be seen that the clinician's expertise is displayed through eliciting and shaping moves that provide a structure for client change (Muntigl & Horvath, 2005). For example, Muntigl and Horvath analyzed psychotherapy sessions from a systemic functional linguistic perspective and stated that through the explicit direction of the interaction, " . . . a narrative therapist's expertise

opens up a space for clients to become better experts of their lives, how problems are influencing their lives and how they may, in turn, influence problems" (pp. 228–229).

Although this chapter has focused on the micro-features associated with therapeutic genres, it is worth considering also the broader issues raised by Fairclough in relation to genre (Fairclough, 2005). This researcher notes that discourse genres are the means by which the activity of governance is conducted—that is, cultural stability and cultural change are inextricably linked with stasis or change within genres. Thus, when speech-language pathologists experience discomfort or hesitancy when changing genres of therapy, this is perhaps best viewed as a signal that the activity of therapy is itself being changed in some way. Such signals provide important opportunities for critical analysis of the purpose and achievement of therapeutic purposes, and for identification of the way forward in the development of effective intervention.

It is not surprising, in view of the foregoing complexities, that mastery of therapeutic genres presents challenges to novices. As noted by Peloquin and Osborne (2003), occupational therapy students often grapple with the challenge of learning to manage the expected discourse demands of the workplace, because their primary experience is gained in tutorials and lectures, which require the development of very different discourse skills. These researchers describe their approach as creating a "practice climate," and the strategies they report are essentially interactive discourse strategies. In lectures, for example, strategies include selecting random responders, demanding full sentence responses, pressing for clarity in answers, expecting active listening (possibly the greatest shift from the lecture genre, which demands passive listening), timing class tasks, springing surprises, imposing ambiguity, inviting disagreement, and giving feedback openly (Peloquin & Osborne, p. 80). These discourse features, which are more commonly associated with workplace environments, are mapped onto the lecture genre and are explicitly discussed with students as ways of learning the discourse of the workplace.

Of course, other spoken discourse types exist besides the ones described in this chapter, in both academic and workplace environments, although broadly speaking, these other ways of communicating tend to be part of more socially generic types of discourse. For example, Swales (2002) suggests that although academic written discourse tends to show distinctive generic patterns for different disciplines, academic spoken discourse appears to be more generically associated with a university community of practice. Also, workplace environments have been characterized by bureaucratic discourse, which reflects and instantiates the hierarchies of power in getting things done within organizations (Harrison & Young, 2004). In both academic and other employment contexts, expert speech-language pathologists will be involved in workshops and conference presentations, and in complex negotiations and formal meetings as part of everyday practice, and an understanding of these broader genres is useful for the development of increasing expertise in these types of discourse.

Possibly one of the biggest surprises that novices experience is that they cannot make assumptions that their expertise gained from other situations will transfer into the new situation. For example, Stillman and colleagues describe the surprise of students that their expertise in interaction with children in general did not carry over into their ability to interact with children with autism spectrum disorders (Stillman, Snow, & Warren, 1999). In Chapter 7, the discussion turns to the consideration of how expertise develops in the discourse of speech-language pathology.

References

Alston, M., Sherratt, S., Ferguson, A., & Vajak, J. (2006). *Outcomes in a chronic aphasia group: Measures and results.* Paper presented at the "Stroke: It's time" 2nd Australasian Nursing and Allied Health Stroke Conference, Sydney, July 6–7.

Bakhtin, M. M. (1986). *Speech genres and other late essays (C. Emerson & M. Holquist, Eds.)* (V. W. McGee, Trans.). Austin, TX: University of Texas Press.

Beaufort, A. (2000). Learning the trade: A social apprenticeship model for gaining writing expertise. *Written Communication, 17*(2), 185–223.

Boone, D. R., & Prescott, T. E. (1972). Content and sequence analyses of speech and hearing therapy. *ASHA, 14,* 58–62.

Brookshire, R. H. (1976). A system for coding and recording events in patient-clinician interactions during aphasia treatment sessions. In R. H. Brookshire (Ed.), *Clinical Aphasiology Conference Proceedings* (pp. 228–240). Minneapolis: BRK.

Buchwald, D., Caralis, P. V., Gany, F., Hardt, E. J., Muecke, M. A., & Putsch, R. W. (1993, April). The medical interview across cultures. *Patient Care,* 141–166.

Byng, S., & Black, M. (1995). What makes a therapy? Some parameters of therapeutic intervention in aphasia. *European Journal of Disorders of Communication, 30*, 303–316.

Christie, F. (1997). Curriculum macrogenres as forms of initiation into a culture. In F. Christie & J. R. Martin (Eds.), *Genre and institutions: Social processes in the workplace and school* (pp. 134–160). London: Cassell.

Duchan, J. F. (1999). Reports written by speech-language pathologists: The role of agenda in constructing client competence (ch.10). In D. Kovarsky, J. F. Duchan, & M. Maxwell (Eds.), *Constructing (in)competence: Disabling evaluations in clinical and social interaction* (pp. 223–224). Mahwah, NJ: Lawrence Erlbaum Associates.

Fairclough, N. (1989). *Language and power.* London: Longman.

Fairclough, N. (2003). Genres and generic structure. In *Analysing discourse* (pp. 65–86). London: Routledge.

Fairclough, N. (2005). Critical discourse analysis in transdisciplinary research. In R. Wodak & P. Chilton (Eds.), *A new agenda in (critical) discourse analysis: Theory, methodology and interdisciplinarity* (pp. 53–70). Amsterdam: John Benjamins.

Ferguson, A. (1998). Analysis of learning interactions. In K. Hird (Ed.), *Expanding horizons: Proceedings of the conference of The Speech Pathology Association of Australia, Fremantle, 11–15 May.* Perth: School of Speech and Hearing Science, Curtin University of Technology.

Ferguson, A. (1999). Clinical Forum: Lead article. Learning in aphasia therapy: It's not so much what you do, but how you do it! *Aphasiology, 13*(2), 125–132, 147–150.

Ferguson, A., & Elliot, N. (2001). Analysing aphasia treatment sessions. *Clinical Linguistics & Phonetics, 15*(3), 229–243.

Fernsten, L. (2005). Discourse and difference. *International Journal of Inclusive Education, 9*(4), 371–387.

Fox, S. A., & Giles, H. (1996). Interability communication: Evaluating patronizing encounters. *Journal of Language and Social Psychology, 15*(3), 265–290.

Grossen, M., & Orvig, A. S. (1998). Clinical interviews as verbal interactions: A multidisciplinary outlook. *Pragmatics, 8*(2), 149–154.

Hagstrom, F., & Wertsch, J. V. (2004). Grounding social identity for professional practice. *Topics in Language Disorders, 24*(3), 162–173.

Hand, L. (2001). Setting the tone: Interviews between speech pathologists and parents of children from non-dominant cultural groups. In L. Wilson & S. Hewat (Eds.), *Evidence and innovation: Proceedings of the 2001 Speech Pathology Australia national conference* (pp. 299–306). Melbourne: Speech Pathology Australia.

Hand, L. (2003). *Discourses in the professional practices of speech pathology interviews.* Unpublished PhD thesis, Macquarie University, Sydney.

Hand, L. (2006). Clinicians as "information givers": What communication access are clients given to speech-language pathology services? *Topics in Language Disorders, 26*(3), 240–265.

Harrison, C., & Young, L. (2004). Bureaucratic discourse: Writing in the "comfort zone." In L. Young & C. Harrison (Eds.), *Systemic functional linguistics and critical discourse analysis* (pp. 231–246). London: Continuum.

Hasan, R. (1985). The structure of a text. In M. A. K. Halliday & R. Hasan (Eds.), *Language, context, and text: Aspects of language in a social-semiotic perspective* (pp. 184–211). Geelong, Victoria, Australia Deakin University Press.

Hasan, R. (1994). Situation and the definition of genres. In A. D. Grimshaw (Ed.), *What's going on here? Complementary studies of professional talk* (Vol. 2 of the *Multiple Analysis Project*). Norwood, NJ: Ablex.

Hein, N., & Wodak, R. (1987). Medical interviews in internal medicine. Some results of an empirical investigation. *Text, 7*(1), 37–65.

Higgs, J., McAllister, L., & Rosenthal, J. (2005). Learning academic writing. In J. Higgs, A. Sefton, A. Street, L. McAllister,

& I. Hay (Eds.), *Communicating in the health and social sciences* (pp. 29–41). Oxford: Oxford University Press.

Hood, S. (2005). What is evaluated, and how, in academic research writing? The co-patterning of attitude and field. *Australian Review of Applied Linguistics, Series S*(19), 23–40.

Horton, S. (2006). A framework for description and analysis of therapy for language impairment in aphasia. *Aphasiology, 20*(6), 528–564.

Horton, S., & Byng, S. (2000). Examining interaction in language therapy. *International Journal of Language & Communication Disorders, 35*(3), 355–375.

Hyland, K. (2005). Stance and engagement: A model of interaction in academic discourse. *Discourse Studies, 7*(2), 173–192.

Kwan, B. S. C. (2006). The schematic structure of literature reviews in doctoral theses of applied linguistics. *English for Specific Purposes, 25*, 30–55.

Kovarsky, D., Kimbarow, M., & Kastner, D. (1999). The construction of incompetence during group therapy with traumatically brain injured adults. In D. Kovarsky, J. F. Duchan & M. Maxwell (Eds.), *Constructing (in)competence: Disabling evaluations in clinical and social interaction* (chap. 13, pp. 291–312). Mahwah, NJ: Lawrence Erlbaum.

Labov, W., & Waletzky, J. (1967). Narrative analysis: Oral versions of personal experience. In J. Helm (Ed.), *Essays on the verbal and visual arts* (pp. 12–44). Seattle: University of Washington Press.

Laufer, E. A., & Glick, J. (1996). Expert and novice differences in cognition and activity: A practical work activity. In Y. Engestrom & D. Middleton (Eds.), *Cognition and communication at work* (pp. 177–198). Cambridge: Cambridge University Press.

Leahy, M. M. (2004). Therapy talk: Analyzing therapeutic discourse. *Language, Speech, and Hearing Services in Schools, 35*, 70–81.

Lewis, M. S., & Hand, L. (1998). The discourse of child language intervention sessions: Are student clinicians following teaching exchanges too closely? In K. Hird (Ed.), *Expanding horizons: Proceedings of the Speech Pathology Australia national conference, Fremantle, WA, May 1998* (pp. 25–34). Melbourne: Speech Pathology Australia.

Markova, I. (1991). Asymmetries in group conversations between a tutor and people with learning difficulties. In I. Markova & K. Foppa (Eds.), *Asymmetries in dialogue* (pp. 221–240). Savage, MD: Barnes & Noble Books.

Martin, J. R. (1997). Analysing genre: Functional parameters. In F. Christie & J. R. Martin (Eds.), *Genre and institutions: Social processes in the workplace and school* (pp. 3–39). London: Cassell.

Muntigl, P., & Horvath, A. (2005). Language, psychotherapy and client change: An interdisciplinary perspective. In R. Wodak & P. Chilton (Eds.), *A new agenda in (critical) discourse analysis: Theory, methodology and interdisciplinarity* (pp. 213–242). Amsterdam: John Benjamins.

Peloquin, S. M., & Osborne, K. A. (2003). Establishing a practice climate in academic settings. *Journal of Allied Health, 32*(2), 78–85.

Rumelhart, D. (1975). Notes on a schema for stories. In D. Bobrow & A. Collins (Eds.), *Representation and understanding: Studies in cognitive science* (pp. 211–236). New York: Academic Press.

Shadden, B. B., & Agan, J. P. (2004). Renegotiation of identity: The social context of aphasia support groups. *Topics in Language Disorders, 24*(3), 174–186.

Sinclair, J. M., & Coulthard, R. M. (1975). *Towards an analysis of discourse: The English used by teachers and pupils.* London: Oxford University Press.

Stillman, R., Snow, C., & Warren, K. (1999). "I used to be good with kids." Encounters between speech-language pathology students and children with pervasive developmental disorders (PDD). In D. Kovarsky, J. F. Duchan, & M. Maxwell (Eds.), *Constructing (in)competence: Dis-*

abling evaluations in clinical and social inter-action (pp. 29–48). Mahwah, NJ: Lawrence Erlbaum Associates.

Swales, J. M. (2003). Is the university a com-munity of practice? In S. Sarangi & T. van Leeuwen (Eds.), *Applied linguistics and communities of practice: Selected papers from the annual meeting of the British Asso-ciation for Applied Linguistics, Cardiff Uni-versity, September 2002* (pp. 203–216). London: Continuum.

ten Have, P. (1991). Talk and institution: A reconsideration of the "asymmetry" of doctor-patient interaction. In D. Boden & D. H. Zimmerman (Eds.), *Talk and social structure* (pp. 138–163). Amsterdam: Polity Press.

Veel, R. (1997). Learning how to mean—scientifically speaking: Apprenticeship into scientific discourse in the secondary school. In F. Christie & J. R. Martin (Eds.), *Genre and institutions: Social processes in the workplace and school* (pp. 161–195). London: Cassell.

Watson, C., & Gallois, C. (2002). Patients' interactions with health providers: A lin-guistic category model approach. *Journal of Language and Social Psychology, 21*(1), 32–52.

West, C. (1984). Medical misfires: Mishear-ings, misgivings and misunderstand-ings in physician-patient dialogues. *Discourse Processes, 7,* 107–134.

Wodak, R. (1996). "What pills are you on now?" Doctors ask, and patients answer. In *Disorders of discourse* (pp. 35–62). Lon-don: Longman.

Woodward-Kron, R. (2002). Academic dis-courses and their discourses of learning: Participants, texts and social practices. In C. N. Candlin (Ed.), *Research and prac-tice in professional discourse* (pp. 499–523). Hong Kong: City University of Hong Kong Press.

Woodward-Kron, R. (2005). The role of genre and embedded genres in tertiary students' writing. *Prospect, 20*(3), 24–41.

Worrall, L., Davidson, B., Hersh, D., Howe, T., Ferguson, A., & Sherratt, S. (2006). *What people with aphasia want: Toward person-centred goal-setting in aphasia reha-bilitation.* Research in progress. Unpub-lished manuscript.

7

Intraprofessional Discourse: Discourse Is Learned

How do novices become experts in speech-language pathology? The previous chapter discussed the types of discourse that are involved in the practice of speech-language pathologists. This chapter asks how facility with these discourses is promoted, and what role discourse itself plays in this facilitation of learning. The focus here is on the interactional processes involved in these discourses; Chapter 8 looks at the structural, institutional discourses associated with these questions in relation to curriculum.

A consideration of some relevant terms that appear in the research and professional literature is an appropriate starting point for discussion. The term *clinical* very much reflects a medical model of professional practice and disciplinary knowledge and often is used in opposition to the term *academic*, setting up a dividing line between theory and practice. Speech-language pathologists working within social models of practice typically find that the term *clinical* does not represent their work, in view of its implications relating to location and process (i.e., room-bound, clinician-controlled). Nor do many

educators see the division between *academic* and *clinical* as useful, because it obscures the role of theory in practice and the role of practice in learning. Other disciplines such as social work tend to use the term *field*, as in *field education* or *field experience*, as the contrasting term, but this too implies separation, suggesting that educative roles are somehow outside the field of practice. More recently, the term *professional* has emerged to replace the term *clinical* and has the advantage of reflecting the societal role without specification of setting or process. In the field of education, the term *supervision* has tended to be used to describe the ways teachers' learning is facilitated by another, and possibly this term has arisen within that discipline as a way of distinguishing it from *education* (of children, for example). *Supervision*, however, carries with it an intrinsic assumption of power and responsibility in the relationship, which may or may not reflect the nature of the relationship. For example, a speech-language pathologist with responsibility for patient care would indeed have the role and responsibility to supervise the work of a student, but a visiting educator would not. In this chapter, the terms *professional education* and *professional experience* are used to describe learning about practice, and the location of that learning is specified separately, for example, in an academic environment or a workplace environment. The term *disciplinary education* is used as a broader term to describe learning and teaching that includes professional education within wider theoretical and disciplinary knowledge, and location of learning again is specified separately. The person providing the experience or education is described as an *educator*, with location separately specified, but this is not to imply that supervisory responsibilities are negated.

Throughout this chapter, in considering learning and teaching in the field, it is worth recognizing the current sociocultural shifts occurring more widely in the world. McCarthy draws attention to the current challenges facing the education of audiologists in the early twenty-first century against the background of the experiences and learning styles of "Generation Y," which typically involve a high level of technological competence and accepted mediation of learning by this means, multitasking, strong team-building and peer-learning, and expectations of immediate and concurrent feedback in the context of learning (McCarthy, 2006).

Learning to Be an Expert

At the novice level, both students and professionals can carry out specified tasks, under various degrees of supervision depending on the complexity of the task and familiarity with the task, and less supervision is required as knowledge and experience accumulate. The development of *expertise*, however, involves more than just this accumulation of knowledge and experience and the ability to undertake tasks independently. As Laufer and Glick (1996) argue, expertise involves a transformation such that rather than being task-focused, the expert is goal-focused—the tasks or activities become a means to an end, rather than an end in themselves. Whereas the learning of the knowledge and skills to do tasks is cognitively mediated, the transformation required for the shift from novice to expert is mediated socioculturally. The novice is standing on the periphery of a community of practice (Wenger, 1998; Wenger, McDermott, & Snyder, 2002), considered as a social group or subculture within society comprising professionals who hold similar goals and values; the transition from novice to expert is one of movement from legitimate peripheral participation (Lave & Wenger, 1991) to assumption of a central role within that community. Learning within this perspective can be seen as "changing patterns of participation in specific social practices within communities of practice" (Gee, 2004, p. 39), and the allied health field is just one such community into which student practitioners are gaining entry (Walker, 2001). Novices entering a community of practice have been seen as entering a cognitive apprenticeship—that is, learning to think like a seasoned practitioner (Brown, Collins, & Duguid, 1989). Learning in this cognitive apprenticeship is seen to be facilitated through scaffolding (such as through modeling and shaping), so Vygotsky's notions of learning occurring within "zones of proximal development" are central here: Learning occurs between the level at which the professional can perform independently and the level at which acceptable performance requires assistance from another (Wertsch, 1985, 2005). Thus, this cognitive apprenticeship is mediated through social means, through the scaffolding provided by the other. This social learning is mediated through discourse and has been explored with reference to learning in the school context by critical linguists working from a systemic functional linguistic perspective (Christie & Martin, 1997). The term "discourse apprenticeship" was coined by Cope (2005, p. 44) to describe this focus on how discourse serves to facilitate social learning within communities of practice, and it is discourse apprenticeship that is the focus of this chapter.

The process of professional socialization into a community of practice is argued to be most powerful in authentic situations. Many ways have been developed to increase the authenticity of learning situations in the academic environment—for example, problem-based learning (Rose, 2005). Feedback from students in a medical problem-based learning program, however, indicated that as students moved into their workplace professional education experiences, they still reported a need to shift their learning style from the logical reasoning approach required in the classroom to a pattern identification approach in the workplace (Prince, Boshuizen, Van der Vleuten, & Scherpbier, 2005). It has been argued that learning experiences can be authentic regardless of setting (Brown et al., 1989), and Cruice posits a "continuum of reality clinical education" (Cruice, 2005, p. 165), such as in the use of simulated patients in academic environments (Edwards, Franke, & McGuiness, 1995).

Many processes contribute to the transformation of the novice to expert, and such processes are described comprehensively in current publications about professional education (L. McAllister & Lincoln, 2004; L. McAllister, Lincoln, McLeod, & Maloney, 1997; Rose & Best, 2005). These transformative processes require the active engagement of the learner, rather than being simply emergent from the accumulation of experience. As Ericsson and Charness (1997) have stated, " . . . individuals improve their performance and attain an expert level, not merely as an automatic consequence of more experience with an activity but rather through structured learning and effortful adaptation" (p. 5).

One of the major processes that shapes the learning of novice students is that of feedback through both formal and informal evaluations. A formal evaluation of student performance is one that is standardized, such as the assessment tasks and marking and grading processes in disciplinary education in academic environments. Formal evaluation of student performance in the workplace environment has been rare in speech-language pathology (and indeed in any related discipline), but validity and reliability have been established for a newly developed tool, COMPASS™, Competency Assessment in Speech Pathology (McAllister, et. al, 2006). This tool's validity arises largely through its embedding of the standards of the community of practice (*Competency based occupational standards for speech pathologists—entry level (revised)*, 2001), as well as from its grounding in the shared understandings with regard to novice-, intermediate-, and entry-level performance indicators researched across educators in the workplace and academic environments and students (S. McAllister, 2005). Of interest, as discussed in Chapter 3, this formal, standardized assessment tool foregrounds the role of formative assessment in learning through its provision of a structure in which informal discursive processes of feedback are embedded within the formal assessment structure. Such embedding of informal processes of evaluation is provided in feedback on student assignments in the academic environment, again embedded within the formal criteria for marking on the assignment. Solely informal processes that allow for evaluative feedback are present in both academic and workplace environments, and the discourse that mediates these informal processes is the focus of the rest of this chapter.

Learning Mediated through Written Discursive Feedback

As discussed in Chapter 6, written discourses in the academic and workplace environments fall within particular genres, which constitute one of the provinces of learning for novices. When students receive written feedback about their written discourse, they typically are receiving feedback about the extent to which their attempts are matching the target genre. Thus, the focus of informal *written feedback* to students on their work in the academic

environment is concerned with style, rather than substance (Crabbe & Lewis, 2002; Lee, 2002). Feedback about the extent to which a student has or has not mastered the genre frequently conflates the extent to which the student's understanding is consistent with the assessor's teaching goal, and the extent to which the student's writing is adequately conveying that understanding within the target genre demands. In view of the interrelationship of thought or schema and language, it should not be surprising that identifying whether the student's problem lies with learning per se or with the expression of learning often is hard for the assessor. Feedback is not impersonal, however; it both reveals the identity of the giver and shapes the identity of the recipient. In considering what in fact this feedback provides, Fernsten (2005) argues that students learn that they are "bad writers" (p. 373), rather than learning ways to think and ways in which writing can express that thinking. Quite possibly, they also learn a lot about the assessor's identity as expert and their inferior status in relation to the wider community of practice (Beaufort, 2000), rather than necessarily learning ways to move from their current understanding to increased understanding. Adopting a critical literacy approach to facilitating the writing of disciplinary discourse would entail explicit teaching of the types of genres, as well as explicit feedback aimed to signal the options and resources in different genres for expressing students' ideas. One of the inherent difficulties associated with written feedback as an interaction between teacher and learner is that it is truncated, consisting of a single-move response to the student's work, with no structural provision for the dialogue to continue. Of course, some students will subsequently discuss their work with the assessor, but these interactions are highly marked for situations of failure—for a majority of students, the assessor as expert has the power of the last word.

New developments and applications of *e-learning* technology have opened up new domains for written discursive feedback, which do allow for greater interactivity. Such developments are being taken up rapidly by the current generation of learners (McCarthy, 2006). The benefits of e-learning from a power perspective are widely recognized as including increased opportunity for all students to contribute, because those who require more time to formulate questions and responses get an opportunity to do this through discussion forum facilities; thus, e-learning is seen as providing greater opportunity for individual interaction between lecturer and students. This increased equity of access is balanced by the downside for socioeconomically disadvantaged students, who may have decreased access to home computers and adequate speed of Internet connection for real-time online participation. The benefits of e-learning depend crucially on how the technology is used, because much of e-learning simply reproduces old discourses in new ways: For example, instead of provision of printed lecture handouts and course readings, students access these on Microsoft Office® PowerPoint slides and Adobe® Portable Document Files (PDF). Both the virtual chat and discussion board facilities, however, offer new options for learning through feedback. Although virtual chat bears many of the discourse markers of

spoken discourse (e.g., turn-taking, informal language, fragmentary utterances), its instantiation in written form provides the opportunity to look back over the discourse generated through the course and reflect on it, which is helpful for both student and educator. Haywood's research indicated that students using virtual chat also carried across spoken features such as open criticism (Haywood, 2004), which provided for peer learning with moderation by the educator. Discussion boards, without the time constraints of virtual chat, tended to elicit discourse features closer to the end-goal academic discourse genre and allowed for an unfolding reiteration of ideas, feedback, and debate. As a point of interest, Haywood found that the students who used an informal register in virtual chat were seen to adopt more professional discourse features in the discussion boards; contrasting the two explicitly with students will provide an opportunity to facilitate critical awareness.

E-learning as a means of professional development in the workplace is just emerging, with barriers identified in terms of the need for skill development, time constraints on preparation and delivery, and the continuing need for face-to-face interaction in learning (Childs, Blenkinsopp, Hall, & Walton, 2005). A foreseeable development is that virtual chat and discussion boards will open up new written discourses for professional discussions in the workplace—ones that will facilitate greater opportunities for feedback about ideas among experts in the field beyond the current e-mail discussion groupings.

Journaling is a type of evaluative written discourse that is used as a process to facilitate learning and development across the continuum of novice to expert (Freeman, 2001). Giving feedback on the written reflections of others, however, is at odds with the aims of self-evaluation and yet arguably is a powerful process for learning. To address this need, Plack and colleagues suggest a coding system to provide feedback to the journal writer, which looks at how the writer is reflecting (e.g., level of abstraction), rather than the content (Plack, Driscoll, Bissett, McKenna, & Plack (2005). In this type of feedback, the educator attempts to facilitate the critical process itself, in order to prompt further reflection and development.

Written feedback also is provided on students' spoken discourse—for instance, on their seminar presentations in the academic environment and on their assessment and therapy interactions in the workplace environment. In the workplace environment, written feedback often is given in parallel with spoken feedback. This latter aspect of feedback is considered next.

Learning Mediated through Spoken Discourse

Expert-Novice Conferencing

In speech-language pathology, the mediation of learning through discussion between the educator and the student (intraprofessional mentoring, or professional supervision) in the workplace often is described as "supervisory conferencing," and much of the literature that guides practice in this area has been based on educational models (McGovern & Dean, 1991). Educational models of supervisory conferencing focus on the teaching of knowledge and skills, and on the provision of corrective feedback to novices regarding their observed performance. Such specific teaching provides a vehicle for a broader agenda, in that it facilitates what Atkinson (1999) describes as "cultural reproduction" (p. 104).

The discussions between medical interns and their preceptors (attending physicians) in a study by Erickson (1999) provide a useful parallel with much of the conferencing between speech-language pathologists and their students: The attending physician has responsibility for the management of the case, but the student is conducting as much of the examination and management as is appropriate for his or her stage of learning. Erickson's particular focus for consideration is how teaching gets done in this interaction, while at the same time how the participants manage the collegial nature of the interaction. The teaching taking place in such interactions is as much about modeling appropriate supervision as it is about the teaching of knowledge and skills—in other words, the cultural reproduction here is about reproducing not only another clinician but also another future educator. Erickson observed that the experts made use of strategies of indirect correction (a feature commonly reported as a face-saving teaching strategy—discussed later in this chapter) but also adopted what Erickson describes as a kind of rhetorical "prolepsis" (p. 120) or anticipation of future competence, analogous to the way parents foster language acquisition through treating unclear utterances as meaningful, rather than correcting all the time. The dilemma is that the expert is still responsible for the management of the case and therefore has to make corrections but at the same time must find ways to accept the contributions of the novice.

A third strategy that Erickson (1999) describes as used by experts is that of finding a point of "co-membership" (p. 114), which enables a more equal footing (Goffman, 1981) between the expert and the novice in their discussions. Erickson suggests that experts do this through explicit discussion of uncertainty in the field of knowledge, which sets up a shared alignment between the expert and the novice in relation to the field—"we are both in this profession." For novices, one of the ways of showing and building co-membership is through the use of in-group expressions and ways of talking. In Erickson's (1999) study, increasing expertise was associated with greater likelihood of switching between use of formal genre conventions of case presentation and medical terms and use of more colloquial registers and terms—use of "bag" for "colostomy bag," for example (Erickson, 1999, p. 123). This strategy can be problematic for novices, because they can be open to judgment of *not* being competent by stepping out of a "professional role" when adopting this discourse feature displayed by experts. As discussed later on, the display of competence through discourse is one of the main sources of judgment regarding the development of expertise.

Such surface features of the discourse reflect a deeper mirroring of the way in which the voice of the learner is transmuted into that of the expert. As Atkinson (1999) notes, the discourse between the expert attending physician and the novice medical intern reflects a similar process to that which occurs between doctors and patients. Medical encounters involve a process whereby the patient's real-world narrative or voice is transmuted into medical discourse, in that the attending physician " . . . interrogates, elicits information, and locates it within a framework of medical knowledge and practice" (Atkinson, p. 99). Supervisory encounters involve a process whereby the novice's narrative of events is transmuted into the professional discourse, through the interrogation and reframing of the expert. Erickson (1999) relates this notion of the appropriation of voice to Bakhtin's ideas of voice and speech genre (Bakhtin, 1986), suggesting that social identity is formed through this process. The novice is still at the periphery of practice and has not yet fully internalized (as in the sense of Vygotsky's notion of inner speech) the professional register (Wertsch, 2005) but is still able to begin participation in the community of practice. Learning occurs through the modeling of the discourse by the expert, followed by matching of that discourse by the novice, with such modeling and matching occurring across the total experience within an authentic workplace setting, not just in formal supervisory conferences. Plack (2006) found that, in a study of physical therapy students, interpersonal and communication skills were reported by students to have been learned not only in clinical interactions but in staff meetings and in the lunch room as well. Plack argues that professional identification (alignment, co-membership) with the community of practice arises out of these experiences in which the learning is tacit, not taught. Such tacit learning takes place, almost incidentally, in the context of the myriad of social interactions and incidents that occur during professional placement experiences in workplace settings. Keppler and Luckmann (1991) examined the way teaching exchanges emerge spontaneously in casual conversations, noting that although participants may open such exchanges through asking questions, those taking on the educator role find ways in which to introduce a teaching moment. These investigators note that such incidental teaching moments are treated as conversational asides, which contrast sharply with instances in which interactants can be seen to jointly construct as the teaching of wisdom. In these latter instances, the person in the role of "wisdom-giver" takes and is allowed extended floor-holding opportunities, and the moment becomes central to the ongoing discourse.

The feature of expert-novice discourse that differentiates it from discussions among peers (discussed later on) is that of the power difference between interactants (Best, 2005). This interactional aspect of expert-novice learning situations may involve any of several types of power. The expert typically has legitimate power in the sense of having been assigned this role institutionally through the recognition of qualifications and experience. This legitimate power often involves the role of assessor, so that the expert has the power of gate-keeping, allowing or disallowing the novice's next steps toward expert status. This assessment role involves the power of rewards given or withheld, and feedback acts as

an interim reward system toward institutional assessment. The expert also has the power of influence, as the referent or model of the role toward which the novice is actively working. It is highly likely that broad sociocultural influences related to power such as gender are likely to play a major role in the learning interactions between experts and novices (McHale & Carr, 1998), but these have been little explored in speech-language pathology or other related fields.

With reference to power and learning interactions in speech-language pathology, Wagner and Hess (1999) looked at the types of power that 61 speech-language pathology educators in the workplace and their students (69 beginners and 69 advanced) perceived to be used by the educators. The perceptions of power were similar for the beginning students and for their educators, but a mismatch was noted in the perceptions of the advanced students and their educators: The educators perceived that they used less power based on their expertise and less power based on their institutional role (legitimate power), and more power associated with positive and negative feedback (reward power) than was perceived by the advanced students. Such mismatches in perception of the power relationship may result in conflict. McCready and colleagues (1996) explored the ways in which speech-language pathologists may respond to conflict in supervisory interactions through looking at their choices from a limited number of set responses to hypothetical conflict scenarios. The speech-language pathology educators selected, in order of frequency, first collaborative, then avoidance, and then competitive (directive) responses, but their choice of response depended on whether the conflict scenario involved personal crisis or an organizational crisis. Essentially, if the educator saw the situation from a professional frame of reference, this prompted a more direct and confrontational response to conflict. McCready and colleagues' study, however, is focused on student compliance as the fault line for conflict and thus is built on the implicit assumption of coercive power within the overt construct of legitimate power. Taken together, these studies by Wagner and Hess and McCready and colleagues point to the need to ask questions about the extent to which learning interactions between speech-language pathology experts and novices are about displaying and perpetuating the power difference, rather than facilitating the movement of the novice toward equal status as expert.

The implicit agenda of experts in educator roles will be shaped not only by their understanding of the power relationship but also by the theoretical framework in relation to facilitation of learning and change that they use in the role as professional with the client. The publicly available video-recorded supervisory conferences of leading experts in psychotherapy with the same supervisee were studied by Holloway, Freund, Gardner, Nelson, and Walker (1989). The analysis of the discourse was based on speech act theory. The interactions observed for these experts in supervisory conference were similar in that they all adopted a teacher-learner role pattern; additionally, however, the study identified discourse patterns that were largely consistent with each expert's theoretical orientation. For example, Albert

Ellis (the originator of rational emotive behavioral therapy) expressed power explicitly in the relationship with prominent use of giving advice, whereas Carl Rogers (the well-known proponent of client-centered therapy) provided encouragement and elicited opinions. This study suggests that educators' "macro" perspectives will influence the "micro"-management of interactions with the student.

Some of these aspects of the discourse involved in the micro-management of the interaction between experts and novices can be seen in Example 7–1, which presents a transcript of an interaction between a speech-language pathology educator (in this case, myself) and a student (Ferguson, 1997).

In this example, the educator responds to what amounts to a request for guidance from the student in turn 1 (" . . . wasn't getting anywhere . . . but you said you'd tried . . . ") with an explicit recognition of uncertainty in the field (" . . . depends . . . why you'd work on it"), thereby aligning the educator and the student in co-membership. The question asked by the educator in turn 2, however, is loaded: In the unfolding discourse, the student does not know if this is a "genuine" question —whether the educator is asking her, as a fellow member of the profession, what she would do—or if the educator is asking her this question as a "test" of her professional thinking. In turn 4, it is apparent that the question at turn 2 was a teaching move because the educator provides feedback ("Right."), rather than simply acknowledging or building on the information given. Supervisory questions can be seen as performing many functions (May, 1989), but one of the main functions is as a

> ## Example 7–1
> ## Questions From the Expert
>
> (*Key:* E, educator; S, student ; < >, overlapping speech.)
>
> (The educator and the student are discussing plans for therapy for a female patient with severe aphasia after traumatic brain injury. This exchange starts at turn 41 of a 336-turn supervisory conference.)
>
> 1   S: Yes, and she was trying so hard and wasn't getting anywhere . . . yeah . . . um . . . what was I going to say . . . um . . . her "yes-no" . . . but you said you'd worked on that and it didn't really . . .
>
> 2   E: Well, it depends what . . . why you'd work on it. Why would you work on it?
>
> 3   S: Oh, because it . . . otherwise it's just "ten," "Joe" [*referring to the perseverative utterances used by the client*] . . .
>
> 4   E: Right.
>
> 5   S: Um . . . you know, because she can understand what you're saying . . .
>
> 6   E   Ah . . .
>
> 7   S: . . . and to have a reliable answer, "yes" or "no," . . . um . . . that . . . that's if she can correctly understand what she's saying. It's really hard to know if she is, or if she's just responding, by saying anything, you know, because she sort of says "yep yep yep yes ten" . . . whatever else she's <chosen.>
>
> 8   E: <Do you> think we know nonverbally whether she means "yes" or "no"? . . . Like forgetting what she says?
>
> 9   S: Um . . . no, I couldn't remember from the session. I was talking to "Ellen " [*another student*] about it before, and I said, maybe if we could get her to gesture, nodding and shaking her head . . .
>
> 10   E: Yes, yes, yes—yeah, I agree.

teaching move, in making suggestions indirectly or in testing learning. In an exchange analysis of such sequences based on systemic functional linguistics (Berry, 1981; O'Donnell, 1991), statements such as those made by the student in turns 1 and 3 are described as semantic moves reflecting the role of "primary knower." When seeking information that is not known, then a person is in the role of "secondary knower." However, when, in a particular move, the fact that the person is in the role of "knower" is not revealed until a subsequent move, then that move is described as a "delayed primary knower" move. The delayed primary knower move thus describes what is going on in such teaching moves, in terms of the way information is shared or withheld. Example 7–1 presents a further delayed primary knower move at turn 8, when the educator speaks ("do you think we know . . . "), and again it is the follow-up move at turn 10 (" . . . yeah, I agree") that reveals the nature of this move. The delayed primary knower sequence is the vehicle for the type of scaffolding through which learning can occur, previously discussed in this chapter—that is, the educator uses the type and level of question and the feedback regarding the response to engage the student in the target professional discourse about reasoning or decision-making. A direct parallel exists between this type of scaffolding through language and that harnessed in therapy for both adults with aphasia (Avent & Austermann, 2003) and children (N. W. Nelson, 2005). Students tacitly learn about scaffolding through their own experience as learners, but from a critical discourse perspective, an important opportunity for students' learning lies in making explicit the discourse scaffolding between student and educator, because awareness opens the opportunity to develop their own skills as future educators and in their work with clients. For example, Shapiro (1994) provides a case example of using the analysis of supervisory conferencing as a means to promote reflection and change in both supervisor and supervisee behavior.

Asking questions in order to facilitate learning performs the function of repair by the "other," and such repair, although uncommon in general conversation (Schegloff, Jefferson, & Sacks, 1977), distinctively marks the learning interactions between experts and novices. "Other" repair typically occurs in the "next turn" position but can occur in later turns (Schegloff, 2000). Example 7–1 also illustrates the power of "other" initiation to prompt self-repair, as in turn 6, when the educator challenges the student's description of the patient's auditory comprehension ("Ah . . . "), which is speedily repaired by the student in turn 7 (" . . . it's really hard to know if she is . . . "). In these ways, the resources of turn-taking provide for the exploitation of question-answer adjacency pairs and repair sequences for the purposes of providing indirect strategies for teaching, through which experts mitigate against the face-threat of criticism and suggestions (Wajnryb, 1998). Such mitigation, however, can render the intended corrective intent of feedback opaque to the novice: For example, in the study by Vasquez (2004) of teachers receiving post-observation supervisor review of their work with students, the teachers perceived that the supervisor had provided little constructive criticism or feedback despite discourse analysis revealing considerable provision of such feedback modulated through the use of positive and negative politeness strategies.

Expert-novice interactions continue to play an important role in professional development throughout the professional's working life. For example, in postgraduate research education, qualified and experienced speech-language pathologists find themselves back in this close supervisory relationship, and similar issues arise in the supervisory process (Rudolph, 1994) in terms of cognitive and social apprenticeship, as mediated through the discourse (spoken and written). Just as with earlier-stage professional learning interactions, postgraduate research supervision involves multiple and intersecting levels of reciprocal expertise. For example, in earlier-stage professional learning interactions, the educator may be younger, with less real-world experience, than a more mature student, and in postgraduate research supervision, the student may bring the greater professional specialist expertise to the relationship. Grant (2003) discusses this multilayered relationship in terms of the different social positioning of the interactants (pp. 182–183) and suggests that previous experiences in the experience and discourse of supervision will play a major role unless critically and explicitly examined. These issues of multiple identities arise in all expert-novice relationships, and Jacoby and Gonzales (1991) argue that it is useful to recognize the expert-novice relationship as dynamic, rather than static. The relationship is dynamic in that novices become experts (and this is the inherent tension in the supervisory power relationship), and in that the relationship is locally negotiated moment by moment in the discourse. As Jacoby and Gonzales describe, a "macro" expert can become a "micro" novice at any moment—for example, in indicating uncertainty and seeking information from others. Indeed, the expert's ability to manage this fluidity is one of the ways of signaling co-membership and of modeling the way experts manage their identity.

Supervisory expertise is developmental, and in one of the few studies of this issue in speech-language pathology, Smith and Anderson (1982b) found that in 45 interactions between 15 supervisor-student pairs, ratings of more indirectness were correlated with more training (professional development workshops on supervision, and hours of coursework beyond a master's degree level). In other words, the types of micro-management skills that have been illustrated and discussed do appear to be related to ongoing development of expertise. Supervisors tend to adjust their supervisory style not only for the stage of the learner but also with stage of experience of supervisor (Stoltenberg, McNeill, & Crethar, 1994). As well as accumulating experience in their cultural contexts, educators are "culturally reproduced"—that is, they learn to educate chiefly from their own experience of being supervised (Rushton & Lindsay, 2003). It is useful to recognize that interactions between more and less expert clinicians (novice-expert, whether student or colleague) are of mutual benefit in terms of learning and socialization, and that novices guide their own instruction through their responsiveness (Wintermantel, 1991). As Avent and Austerman (2003) describe in their application of "reciprocal scaffolding treatment," the expert scaffolds the novice's learning through the discourse, but at the same time, the novice, through questions and responsiveness, scaffolds the expert's understanding and discovery of knowledge. Thus, the joint experience is itself creating socialization for both—for the novice to become a speech-language pathologist but also for the expert in understanding his or her identity as both speech-language pathologist (expert clinician) and educator. The tacit nature of this learning means that reflective practice offers educators an important tool to "unpack" their theoretical assumptions about learning and power and to consider how these may influence how they go about the business of facilitating the movement of novices from the periphery to the center of practice.

The socialization aspect of professional education is both powerful and dangerous—socialization can start to look very like homogenization without a critical perspective. This apparent paradox is well delineated by Cope, who in an overview of the area notes that traditional apprenticeship and cognitive apprenticeship models are essentially about conformity, that is, reproducing required skills for the workplace (Cope, 2005). For example, systemic functional linguistic theorists in line with Bernstein (1996) point to the way in which the education system is stratified to provide the social strata of the community, resulting in a mirroring of the levels in workplace and in education (i.e., basic schooling associated with providing laborers, more advanced schooling associated with providing technical workers, and tertiary education associated with providing professionals). In one sense, however, this sort of stratification can be considered to be dysfunctional for society: While maintaining social order, the constraints on innovation and critical thinking reduce the capacity of a community to adapt to new demands. A micro-example of the dangers of socialization toward conformity can be seen in the study by Lingard, Reznick, DeVito, and Espin (2002), who looked at how professionals within the same discipline talked about professionals in another discipline in discussions about conflict scenarios that were drawn from previous ethnographic research in

operating room interactions. The two disciplines involved were surgical (surgical trainees and surgeons), and nurses. Participants from both disciplines tended to simplify and distort the roles of the other discipline and evidenced very different perceptions and attributions of motivation and responsibility for things said and done in the scenarios (which naturally raises barriers to interdisciplinary practice; refer to Chapter 5). Particularly striking, however, was the finding that the surgical trainees' responses both reflected and were more extreme than the responses of their same-discipline expert. In this situation, novice socialization appeared to be powerfully influenced by expert modeling, and their processes of identity formation meant that novices in fact drew sharper territorial boundaries than those recognized by experts (Lingard et al., 2002). This recognition of the power of professional experience in the workplace for socialization within a discipline raises the question of how educators can promote and critically challenge socialization simultaneously. One way forward in this regard is through the possibilities opened by peer learning, discussed next.

Peer Conferencing

The current generation of learners have extensive experience in learning and problem-solving in teams, because much of their early education has made use of this way of scaffolding learning (McCarthy, 2006), so peer learning for this generation is an expectation, rather than an additional experience. The notion of peer learning involves a range of understandings regarding the extent to which learners can, in fact, be similar—some peer learning, for example, may involve interaction between more experienced and less experienced novices. The essential feature to consider, however, is the extent of the difference in legitimate power between learners (for example, typically a peer would not be assessing the other for the purpose of institutional grading). It is likely that interpersonal power dynamics will play a major role between peers such that feedback may hold social rewards and act as an influence or motivator, and referent power may promote modeling. Much of focus on peer learning has focused on these aspects of interpersonal power as the explanatory force behind why peer learning might be a powerful educative tool; in other words, peer pressure becomes the driving force toward conformity. Sawchuk (2003), however, argues that peer learning offers powerful informal learning opportunities for innovation and critical thinking, precisely because of the lack of power difference. Sawchuk used conversation analysis to investigate the discourse of two computer students working to understand a particular operation of software. This researcher found that the discourse differed in significant ways from typical pedagogical discourse in that the two peers shared in the turn allocation and in that the typical initiation-response-feedback cycle was lacking. Instead, he argued that the students were jointly constructing a "zone of proximal development" in which learning was occurring. He suggests that this sort of learning is potentially political in that expert-

novice learning is about reproduction of the social order (in the sense of Foucault's notion of social order), whereas informal peer learning has potential to be transformative, rather than reproductive.

One way in which this transformative process can be observed is in a transcribed segment of peer learning discourse: In Example 7–2, the same student as in Example 7–1 is now talking with a peer about the same patient. The peer (S2) is asking questions and in a structural sense is taking the role of supervisor in an extended question-answer sequence—for example, asking questions at turns 3, 11, and 19 about the patient's spontaneous production, comprehension, and written production. These questions are not teaching moves, however, because the peer simply accepts the information provided, with comments indicating support for the level of difficulty faced in planning at turns 5, 7, and 13. The closest that the peer comes to evaluative feedback similar to that associated with the expert supervisory role is the affirmation in turn 9 regarding the importance of the student's decision to work on gesture. Of note, however, equivalent learning is evidenced in this peer interaction in Example 7–2, as also seen in the expert-novice interaction in Example 7–1; clearly, the student (S1 in Example 7–2) arrives at an understanding and a plan for action in both exchanges.

The larger set of data from which these samples are drawn derive from three conferences between the educator (myself) and three students, each of whom participated in two conferences with their peers, for a total of nine conference (three expert-novice confer-

Example 7–2
Peer Questions

(*Key:* S1, student 1; S2, student 2.)

(Student 1 and student 2 are midway through their first educational work-place assignment for adult neurological disorders and are discussing plans for therapy for a female patient with severe aphasia after traumatic brain injury. This exchange starts at turn 44 of a 117-turn peer conference.)

1	S2:	I know you've told me she perseverates heaps and heaps.
2	S1:	Yep.
3	S2:	What . . . what does she say, like . . . spontaneously?
4	S1:	"Joe," "twelve," "which one," "not me," "me good, me good," "good for me, good for me."
5	S2:	That's it.
6	S1:	That's it . . . um . . . .Very, very, very rarely, like . . . um . . . I've heard it about four times . . . in two or three sessions. Does she say something that's in context?. She told me . . . she didn't . . . "I don't know." She said "bye bye."
7	S2:	Ooh.
8	S1:	What we want to do is . . . .Well, like . . . what one of my aims is . . . to her to gesture "yes" and "no" correctly.
9	S2:	Yeah—that's a fairly important one.
10	S1:	Yep. But how to do that . . . .
11	S2:	Yeah. You were saying her comprehension's what . . . so-so?
12	S1:	Yeah—it's a bit iffy. You're not sure actually if she's under-standing you, because . . . she can't give you a positive "yes" . . . because . . . "yes" is sort of just like jargon to her.
13	S2:	Ah huh . . . she's a challenge! [*laughs*] [*Turns 14 to 18 omitted*]
19	S2:	So . . . if her . . . .How's her written . . . um . . . .To what extent could she use that?
20	S1:	Write yes and no?
21	S2:	Mm.
22	S1:	I don't know . . . that's a good one. I haven't asked her to do that. We could do . . . she could respond . . .

ences and six peer conferences). The pattern that emerged from an exchange analysis based on systemic functional linguistics (Berry, 1981; O'Donnell, 1991) across these conferences reflected key differences in the use of delayed primary knower moves, with this move associated only with the expert-novice conferences. Analysis of the peer conferences demonstrated a high proportion of questions (secondary knower moves) on the part of the peer who was not working directly with the case being discussed, but an equal balance between the students of information sharing (primary knower moves). By contrast, in the expert-novice conferences, the students asked fewer questions (secondary knower moves), instead tending to put information forward in primary knower moves e.g. making a statement which provided an opportunity for the educator to comment upon rather than directly seeking information. In these expert-novice conferences, the educator took up the greater proportion of information giving (primary knower moves) (Ferguson, 1997).

For experts too, peer learning can offer a powerful means through which change can occur. Titchen (2001) proposes a model for "critical companionship" (p. 80), through which expert professionals can obtain a source of feedback and stimulation toward development of theoretical understandings and practice, in the context of high levels of interpersonal support. Although professional supervision is structured within most workplaces, and the notion of mentorship has some currency in the profession, little is known about the interactive learning processes that are involved in such expert-expert relationships, and how such relationships mediate learning.

For novices, peer learning through discussion takes place throughout placements in which more than one student is involved (Dowling, 1983), although the informal nature of the discussions may mean that this form of learning may be relatively devalued. On the one hand, the lack of power in the relationship between peers provides for opportunities to take risks in discussing learning, and the re-telling of narratives associated with the learning experience performs an important function in identity building (Cortazzi, Jin, Wall, & Cavendish, 2001). On the other hand, in contrast with supervisory conferences, peer conferences carry no opportunity to display competence for the purposes of assessment and this point is explored further in the next section.

Language and Competence

The work of speech-language pathology requires linguistic proficiency of a high order, both in terms of the understanding and production of spoken and written language and also in terms of the metalinguistic understandings and analysis of the communication of others. Beyond that level of proficiency is the relationship between linguistic processing and expertise. The work of Leon and Perez (2001) has shown that experts are better and faster than novices at processing clinically related information presented online in order to form a clinical diagnosis. The novices—in this case, psychology students —tended to be slower and to process information acquired offline (information presented in auditory and written-mode reaction time experiments). In other words, the background knowledge differences between experts and novices affect on-the-spot decision-making capability—novices need more time. Beyond this issue, however, is the additional role that communicative competence plays in mediating clinical competence, and in mediating the judgments of clinical competence.

Communicative Competence and Clinical Competence

Communication skills are integral to clinical competence in student speech-language pathologists. In COMPASS™ (McAllister et al., 2006), communication skills are seen as generic skills underpinning the development of specific professional competencies across all populations and types of disorder. The degree to which communication skills are taught explicitly in both academic and workplace settings appears, anecdotally, to be highly variable. Students in medical programs have received more attention in this regard, perhaps because they have been identified as an at-risk group for failure to develop the communication skills needed for fully effective clinical practice (Royston, 1997). Regardless of the extent to which such skills are taught explicitly, communication typically is a major feature of any assessment of clinical competence. Educators in both professional and academic environments use their observations of the communication of students as a means to assess both their communication skills and their clinical competence. Of interest, in view of the debates around formal and informal assessments of the communication skills of people with communication disorders (refer to Chapters 2 and 3), the methods of assessing students' communication skills are overwhelmingly informal. As previously discussed, informal assessment can be argued to be more valid, yet an equal need exists for infor-

mal assessments to be explicit and systematic—features that are noticably lacking in the means by which the communication skills of speech-language pathology students are assessed.

Even less acknowledged is the extent to which educators (necessarily) rely on the way students talk about their understandings to infer clinical competence. Erickson (1999) discusses this phenomenon in relation to medical interns in discussions with the attending physician. Erickson notes the contradiction faced by the novice in trying to appear fully competent while clearly not yet fully competent (as indicated by continued supervision) (p. 112). These interactions and between the expert and the novice are characterized as occurring "back-stage" by Sarangi and Roberts (1999), in contrast with the encounter with the patient, which is on-stage or "front-stage". For the student, however, both such interactions are on-stage, because their performance is being evaluated at all times, which may explain some of the anxiety reported to be associated with student learning (Chan, Carter, & McAllister, 1994). Students are learning the professional discourses of speech-language pathology (Ferguson & Armstrong, 2004; Pillay, 2001) for both on-stage and back-stage performance.

Part of this communicative competence involves the ability of the student to manage and negotiate the supervisory relationship itself. As Waite (1993) discusses in an ethnographic study of teacher supervision, conversation analysis revealed that some students were able to shape supervisor feedback and to manage adversarial roles without confrontation. Waite stresses that supervision is not a one-way process directed by educator: Students can influence the course that discussions will take in conference and co-construct the perception of their professional competence.

Not all students, however, have these communication skills within their work with clients or with their educators, and those coming from different cultural and linguistic backgrounds face particular challenges.

Cultural and Linguistic Difference and Clinical Competence

Probably the biggest issue for students from cultural and linguistic backgrounds that differ from those of their educators is that the nature and extent of the linguistic-communicative competence required for practice of speech-language pathology are simultaneously undefined and assumed (Clarke, 2005). Students providing speech-language pathology services or talking about their provision of speech-language pathology services in their second language face the situation of not knowing the exact nature of the hurdles—or, to continue the analogy, how high they have to jump. For example, is 100% speech intelligibility required of the student at all times for all clients? (After all, the educator may be seen to need to repeat and clarify information for clients.) Is exact conformity with the grammatical formulations of the educator required? (Many clients may use registers that more closely resemble that of the student than that of the educator.) Despite the lack of definition of just what is needed for either learning or practicing, most speech-language education programs have in place some kind of

gate-keeping mechanism (often prescribed by the educational institution as a whole) that uses prescribed standardized testing designed to preclude entry on the basis of some level of unacceptability (variously specified). As Shohamy (2001) has noted, these language proficiency tests are widely accepted as valid, despite considerable deficiencies in their content and construct validity. "How crucial the knowledge of language is for academic success is still an open question that does not have empirical answers. Yet, language testers determine cut-off scores and thus pretend to know the correct answer and often inform those responsible for admission what score is required" (Shohamy, p. 123).

Thus far, the cultural or linguistic difference of the student has been defined in relation to the educator, not the client. This reference point is deliberately chosen, because within the community of practice, an unexamined assumption is that provision of satisfactory client services depends solely on some assessed level of proficiency of an accredited provider. Accordingly, a student speaking a second language in providing services to a client may be at risk for "clinical incompetence." The question that is *not* asked is whether a qualified speech-language pathologist is providing anything other than competent services to clients who speak another language. Students speaking other languages or even students speaking the same language but from a different culture (Clarke & Quaglio, 2002) tend to become part of a perceived problem; indeed, research indicates that for these students, the learning situation is less than ideal (Marshall, Goldbart, & Evans, 2004). By contrast, visits of students who speak English as a first language to provide services in other countries in which English is not the dominant language are seen as valuable experiences for the native English speakers in increasing their cultural sensitivity, but the value of such visits has been unquestioned with regard to either services provided or colonization of Western cultural values in the field (Trembath, Wales, & Balandin, 2005). As discussed in Chapter 5, provision of services to clients via interpreters is an important yet complex mode of service delivery, and one that is fully accepted within the profession, despite its obvious limitations. As commonly argued within the profession, however, one answer to improved service delivery for clients who speak another language is the greater availability of speech-language pathologists who themselves speak another language. To this end, more students from diverse cultural and linguistic backgrounds need to be taken into to education programs—yet these students often are barred through, first, social and educational disadvantage associated with more general societal disadvantages; second, language gate-keeping requirements; and third, the failure to recognize the need for ways in which both communicative-linguistic competence and clinical competence can codevelop. In this chapter, the role of the educator in socialization to the culture of speech-language pathology has been highlighted, and this recognition of the educator role as cultural guide can be seen to apply to all students across all linguistic and cultural backgrounds (Remedios & Webb, 2005). The need to recognize cultural and linguistic diversity in professional practice as

a widespread phenomenon is pointed out by Pickering and McAllister (2000), who suggest three main guiding concepts to assist this recognition process: the need to move from ethnocentricity to a view of "ethnorelativism," being comfortable with coexisting multiple perspectives, and understanding the discourse systems involved (through understanding the cultural ideology as expressed in the discourse, and through understanding the negotiation of meaning within discourse as central to all discourse) (Pickering, 2005; Pickering & McAllister, 2000).

Bridging the Gap between Theory and Practice

One of the most commonly discussed challenges for professional education is that of narrowing or crossing the gap between theory and practice. This issue goes deeper than matters of whether or not particular theories that are being taught in the classroom are observed by students when they undertake clinical education placements in the workplace (R. Nelson & Ball, 2003). The student in an education program while on professional education placement in the workplace is trying to learn to participate in two different discourses simultaneously. Although the student in the educating organization is being asked to be an independent learner, the pressure of application in the here and now sends a different message. For example, Lincoln and colleagues discuss time management as a stress factor in workplace education (Lincoln, Adamson, & Covic, 2004) and point out the differences between demands on time management in the academic and the workplace environments. In the academic environment, commitments are known well in advance and rarely change, whereas in the workplace environment, commitments need to be responsive to organizational demands (caseload and administrative fluctuations). The difference between the institutional discourses is between the construction of the student's identity as competent in controlled conditions with high independence (educating institution) and as competent in being adaptable in conditions outside the person's control with high interdependence (employing institution). This challenge of dealing with two different discourses is possibly another contributor to the anxiety experienced by students in professional educational work placements: In the research of Chan and colleagues, it was found that although all students reported some degree of anxiety, novice students were anxious about matters such as diagnosis, whereas final-year students' anxiety was related to amount of control (Chan et al., 1994).

In this chapter, a number of bridges have been identified that provide ways in which educators and students can facilitate the learning of these two discourses: formal and informal expert-novice and peer conferencing (whether in academic or workplace environments); journaling; and e-learning discussion boards. Also, explicit teaching of the genres of therapy and of the key aspects known to arise in expert-novice and peer learning interactions offers both the student and the educator opportunities to reflect on the practice of others and themselves (Culatta & Seltzer, 1976; Horton, Byng, Bunning,

& Pring, 2004; Smith & Anderson, 1982a, 1982b). In the next chapter, the differences between the discourses of the educating and employing institutions are explored in relation to issues in curriculum development and the transition of the student to the workplace.

References

Atkinson, P. (1999). Medical discourse, evidentiality and the construction of professional responsibility. In S. Sarangi & C. Roberts (Eds.), *Talk, work and institutional order: Discourse in medical, mediation and management settings* (pp. 75–107). Berlin: Mouton de Gruyter.

Avent, J. R., & Austermann, S. (2003). Reciprocal scaffolding: A context for communication treatment in aphasia. *Aphasiology, 17*(4), 397–404.

Bakhtin, M. M. (1986). *Speech genres and other late essays (C. Emerson & M. Holquist, Eds)* (V. W. McGee, Trans.). Austin, TX: University of Texas Press.

Beaufort, A. (2000). Learning the trade: A social apprenticeship model for gaining writing expertise. *Written Communication, 17*(2), 185–223.

Bernstein, B. (1996). *Pedagogy, symbolic control, and identity: Theory, research, critique*. London: Taylor & Francis.

Berry, M. (1981). Systemic linguistics and discourse analysis: A multi-layered approach to exchange structure. In R. M. Coulthard & M. M. Montgomery (Eds.), *Studies in discourse analysis* (pp. 120–145). London: Routledge & Kegan Paul.

Best, D. (2005). Power issues in clinical education. In M. Rose, D. Best, & J. Higgs (Eds.), *Transforming practice through clinical education, professional supervision and mentoring* (pp. 197–205). Edinburgh: Elsevier Churchill Livingstone.

Brown, J. S., Collins, A., & Duguid, P. (1989, Jan-Feb). Situated cognition and the culture of learning. *Educational Researcher*, 32–42.

Chan, J., Carter, S., & McAllister, L. (1994). Contributions to anxiety in clinical education in undergraduate speech-language pathology students. *Australian Journal of Human Communication Disorders*, 22(1), 57–73.

Childs, S., Blenkinsopp, E., Hall, A., & Walton, G. (2005). Effective e-learning for health professionals and students—barriers and their solutions. A systematic review of the literature—findings from the HeXL project. *Health Information and Libraries Journal*, 22(Suppl. 2), 20–32.

Christie, F., & Martin, J. R. (Eds.). (1997). *Genre and institutions: Social processes in the workplace and school*. London: Cassell.

Clarke, L. (2005). *Competence and diversity: Inclusive strategies for supporting students from non-English speaking backgrounds in speech pathology training programs*. Paper presented at the Speech Pathology Australia national conference, Canberra, May 29–June 2.

Clarke, L., & Quaglio, M. (2002). *A world of English: Issues for speech pathology in Australia*. Paper presented at the Speech Pathology Australia national conference, Alice Springs, Australia, May 20–23.

Competency based occupational standards for speech pathologists—entry level (revised). (2001). Melbourne,Victoria, Australia: Speech Pathology Australia.

Cope, N. (2005). Apprenticeship reinvented: Cognition, discourse and implications for academic literacy. *Prospect*, 20(3), 42–62.

Cortazzi, M., Jin, L., Wall, D., & Cavendish, S. (2001). Sharing learning through narrative communication. *International Journal of Language & Communication Disorders*, 36(Suppl.), 252–257.

Crabbe, D., & Lewis, M. (2002). Towards standards of feedback on written assignments in language teacher education. *Australian Review of Applied Linguistics*, 25(1), 41–51.

Cruice, M. (2005). Common issues but alternative solutions and innovations. *Advances in Speech-Language Pathology*, 7(3), 162–166.

Culatta, R., & Seltzer, H. (1976, Jan). Content and sequence analysis of the supervisory session. *ASHA*, 8–12.

Dowling, S. (1983). Teaching clinic conference participant interaction. *Journal of Communication Disorders*, 16, 385–397.

Edwards, H., Franke, M., & McGuiness, B. (1995). Using simulated patients to teach clinical reasoning. In J. Higgs & M. Jones (Eds.), *Clinical reasoning in the health professions* (pp. 269–278). Oxford: Butterworth-Heinemann.

Erickson, F. (1999). Appropriation of voice and presentation of self as a fellow physician: Aspects of a discourse of apprenticeship in medicine. In S. Sarangi & C. Roberts (Eds.), *Talk, work and institutional order: Discourse in medical, mediation and management settings* (pp. 109–143). Berlin: Mouton de Gruyter.

Ericsson, K. A., & Charness, N. (1997). Cognitive and developmental factors in expert performance (ch.1). In P. J. Feltovich, K. M. Ford, & R. R. Hoffman (Eds.), *Expertise in context: Human and machine* (pp. 3–41). Menlo Park, CA: AAAI Press/MIT Press.

Ferguson, A. (1997). *Knowing and learning in peer conferencing*. Paper presented at the annual national conference of The Speech Pathology Association of Australia, Canberra, Melbourne, March 10–14.

Ferguson, A., & Armstrong, E. (2004). Reflections on speech-language therapists' talk: Implications for clinical practice and education. *International Journal of Language & Communication Disorders*, 39(4), 469–477.

Fernsten, L. (2005). Discourse and difference. *International Journal of Inclusive Education*, 9(4), 371–387.

Freeman, M. (2001). Reflective logs: An aid to clinical teaching and learning. *International Journal of Language & Communication Disorders*, 36(Suppl.), 411–416.

Gee, J. P. (2004). Discourse analysis: What makes it critical? In R. Rogers (Ed.), *An introduction to critical discourse analysis in education* (pp. 19–50). Mahwah, NJ: Lawrence Erlbaum Associates.

Goffman, E. (1981). *Forms of talk.* Oxford: Basil Blackwell.

Grant, B. (2003). Mapping the pleasures and risks of supervision. *Discourse: Studies in the cultural politics of education, 24*(2), 175–190.

Haywood, L. M. (2004). Integrating web-enhanced instruction into a research methods course: Examination of student experiences and perceived learning. *Journal of Physical Therapy Education, 18*(2), 54–65.

Holloway, E. L., Freund, R. D., Gardner, S. L., Nelson, M. L., & Walker, B. R. (1989). Relation of power and involvement to theoretical orientation in supervision: An analysis of discourse. *Journal of Counseling Psychology, 36*(1), 88–102.

Horton, S., Byng, S., Bunning, K., & Pring, T. (2004). Teaching and learning speech and language therapy skills: The effectiveness of classroom as clinic in speech and language therapy student education. *International Journal of Language & Communication Disorders, 39*(3), 365–390.

Jacoby, S., & Gonzales, P. (1991). The constitution of expert-novice in scientific discourse. *Issues in Applied Linguistics, 2*(2), 149–181.

Keppler, A., & Luckman, T. (1991). "Teaching": Conversational transmission of knowledge. In I. Markova & K. Foppa (Eds.), *Asymmetries in dialogue* (pp. 143–165). Savage, MD: Barnes & Noble Books.

Laufer, E. A., & Glick, J. (1996). Expert and novice differences in cognition and activity: A practical work activity. In Y. Engestrom & D. Middleton (Eds.), *Cognition and communication at work* (pp. 177–198). Cambridge: Cambridge University Press.

Lave, J., & Wenger, E. (1991). *Situated learning: Legitimate peripheral participation.* New York: Cambridge University Press.

Lee, J. (2002). Attitudes towards disputable usages among Australian teachers and students. *Australian Review of Applied Linguistics, 25*(1), 109–129.

Leon, J. A., & Perez, O. (2001). The influence of prior knowledge on the time course of clinical diagnosis inferences: A comparison of experts and novices. *Discourse Processes, 31*(2), 187–213.

Lincoln, M., Adamson, B., & Covic, T. (2004). Perceptions of stress, time management and coping strategies of speech pathology students on clinical placement. *Advances in Speech-Language Pathology, 6*(2), 91–99.

Lingard, L., Reznick, R., DeVito, I., & Espin, S. (2002). Forming professional identities on the health care team: Discursive constructions of the "other" in the operating room. *Medical Education, 36*, 728–734.

Marshall, J., Goldbart, J., & Evans, R. (2004). International students of speech and language therapy in the UK: Do we meet their needs? *International Journal of Language & Communication Disorders, 39*(2), 269–284.

May, J. D. (1989). Questions as suggestions: The pragmatics of interrogative speech. *Language & Communication, 9*(4), 227–243.

McAllister, L., & Lincoln, M. (2004). *Clinical education in speech-language pathology.* London: Whurr.

McAllister, L., Lincoln, M., McLeod, S., & Maloney, D. (1997). *Facilitating learning in clinical settings.* Cheltenham, UK: Stanley Thornes.

McAllister, S. (2005). *Competency based assessment of speech pathology students' performance in the workplace.* Unpublished PhD thesis, University of Sydney, Sydney.

McAllister, S. M., Lincoln, M., Ferguson, A., & McAllister, L. (2006). *COMPASS™ (competency assessment in speech pathology) assessment and resource manual.* Melbourne, Victoria, Australia: Speech Pathology Australia.

McCarthy, P. (2006). Clinical education in audiology: The challenge of change. *Seminars in Hearing, 27*, 79–85.

McCready, V., Roberts, J. E., Bengala, D., Harris, H., Kingsley, G., & Krikorian, C.

(1996). A comparison of conflict tactics in the supervisory process. *Journal of Speech and Hearing Research, 39,* 191–199.

McGovern, M. A., & Dean, E. C. (1991). Clinical education: The supervisory process. *British Journal of Disorders of Communication, 26*(3), 373–381.

McHale, E., & Carr, A. (1998). The effect of supervisor and trainee therapist gender on supervision discourse. *Journal of Family Therapy, 20,* 395–411.

Nelson, N. W. (2005). The context of discourse difficulty in classroom and clinic: An update. *Topics in Language Disorders, 25*(4), 322–331.

Nelson, R., & Ball, M. J. (2003). Models of phonology in the education of speech-language pathologists. *Clinical Linguistics & Phonetics, 17*(4–5), 403–409.

O'Donnell, M. (1991). A dynamic model of exchange. *Word, 4,* 293–328.

Pickering, M. (2005). Issues and innovations in clinical education: A view from the USA. *Advances in Speech-Language Pathology, 7*(3), 167–169.

Pickering, M., & McAllister, L. (2000). A conceptual framework for linking and guiding domestic cross-cultural and international practice in speech-language pathology. *Advances in Speech-Language Pathology, 2*(2), 93–106.

Pillay, M. (2001). "Do you speak practice-ese?" A discourse of practice for sharing communication. *International Journal of Language & Communication Disorders, 36*(Suppl), 351–356.

Plack, M. M. (2006). The development of communication skills, interpersonal skills, and a professional identity within a community of practice. *Journal of Physical Therapy Education, 20*(1), 37–46.

Plack, M. M., Driscoll, M., Blissett, S., McKenna, R., & Plack, T. P. (2005). A method for assessing reflective journal writing. *Journal of Allied Health, 34*(4), 199–208.

Prince, K. J. A., Boshuizen, H. P. A., Van der Vleuten, C. P. M., & Scherpbier, A. J. J. A. (2005). Students' opinions about their preparation for clinical practice. *Medical Education, 39,* 704–712.

Remedios, L., & Webb, G. (2005). Clinical educators as cultural guides. In M. Rose & D. Best (Eds.), *Transforming practice through clinical education, professional supervision and mentoring* (pp. 207–218). Edinburgh: Elsevier Churchill Livingstone.

Rose, M., & Best, D. (Eds.). (2005). *Transforming practice through clinical education, professional supervision and mentoring.* Edinburgh: Elsevier Churchill Livingstone.

Rose, M. L. (2005). The cycle of crisis in clinical education: Why national-level strategies must be prioritized. *Advances in Speech-Language Pathology, 7*(3), 158–161.

Royston, V. (1997). How do medical students learn to communicate with patients? A study of fourth-year medical students' attitudes to doctor-patient communication. *Medical Teacher, 19*(4), 257–262.

Rudolph, D. E. (1994). Constructing an apprenticeship with discourse strategies: Professor-graduate student discourse. *Language in Society, 23,* 199–230.

Rushton, A., & Lindsay, G. (2003). Clinical education: A critical analysis using soft systems methodology. *International Journal of Therapy and Rehabilitation, 10*(6), 271–280.

Sarangi, S., & Roberts, C. (1999). The dynamics of interactional and institutional orders in work-related settings. In S. Sarangi & C. Roberts (Eds.), *Talk, work and institutional order: Discourse in medical, mediation and management settings* (pp. 1–57). Berlin: Mouton de Gruyter.

Sawchuk, P. H. (2003). Informal learning as a speech-exchange system: Implications for knowledge production, power and social transformation. *Discourse & Society, 14*(3), 291–307.

Schegloff, E. A. (2000). When "others" initiate repair. *Applied Linguistics, 21*(2), 205–243.

Schegloff, E. A., Jefferson, G., & Sacks, H. (1977). The preference for self-correction in the organization of repair in conversation. *Language, 53,* 361–382.

Shapiro, D. A. (1994). Interaction analysis and self-study: A single-case comparison of four methods of analyzing supervisory conferences. *Language, Speech, and Hearing Services in Schools, 25*, 67–75.

Shohamy, E. (2001). *The power of tests: A critical perspective on the uses of language tests.* Harlow, UK: Pearson Education.

Smith, K. J., & Anderson, J. L. (1982a). Development and validation of an individual supervisory conference rating scale for use in speech-language pathology. *Journal of Speech & Hearing Research, 25*(2), 243–251.

Smith, K. J., & Anderson, J. L. (1982b). Relationship of perceived effectiveness to verbal interaction/content variables in supervisory conferences in speech-language pathology. *Journal of Speech and Hearing Research, 25* (2), 252–261.

Stoltenberg, C. D., McNeill, B. W., & Crethar, H. C. (1994). Changes in supervision as counselors and therapists gain experience: A review. *Professional Psychology: Research and Practice, 25*(4), 416–449.

Titchen, A. (2001). Critical companionship: A conceptual framework for developing expertise. In J. Higgs & A. Titchen (Eds.), *Practice knowledge and expertise in the health professions* (pp. 80–90). Oxford: Butterworth Heinemann.

Trembath, D., Wales, S., & Balandin, S. (2005). Challenges for undergraduate speech pathology students undertaking cross-cultural clinical placements. *International Journal of Language & Communication Disorders, 40*(1), 83–98.

Vasquez, C. (2004). "Very carefully managed": Advice and suggestions in post-observation meetings. *Linguistics and Education, 15*, 33–58.

Wagner, B. T., & Hess, C. W. (1999). Supervisors' use of social power with graduate supervisees in speech-language pathology. *Journal of Communication Disorders, 32*, 351–368.

Waite, D. (1993). Teachers in conference: A qualitative study of teacher-supervisor face-to-face interactions. *American Educational Research Journal, 30*(4), 675–702.

Wajnryb, R. (1998). Telling it like it isn't—exploring an instance of pragmatic ambivalence in supervisory discourse. *Journal of Pragmatics, 29*, 531–544.

Walker, R. (2001). Social and cultural perspectives on professional knowledge and expertise. In J. Higgs & A. Titchen (Eds.), *Practice knowledge and expertise in the health professions* (pp. 22–28). Oxford: Butterworth-Heinemann.

Wenger, E. (1998). *Communities of practice: Learning, meaning, and identity.* Cambridge: Cambridge University Press.

Wenger, E., McDermott, R., & Snyder, W. M. (2002). *Cultivating communities of practice: A guide to managing knowledge.* Boston: Harvard Business School Press.

Wertsch, J. V. (1985). *Vygotsky and the social formation of mind.* Cambridge, MA: Harvard University Press.

Wertsch, J. V. (2005). Vygotsky's two approaches to mediation. In S. Norris & R. H. Jones (Eds.), *Discourse in action: Introducing mediated discourse analysis* (pp. 52–61). London: Routledge.

Wintermantel, M. (1991). Dialogue between expert and novice: On difference in knowledge and their reduction. In I. Markova & K. Foppa (Eds.), *Asymmetries in dialogue* (pp. 124–142). Savage, MD: Barnes & Noble Books.

8

Curriculum Development: Discourse Is Institutionally Based

In this chapter, models and frameworks for curriculum development in speech-language pathology within institutional and wider cultural contexts are discussed and critiqued from a critical discourse perspective. What is taught in speech-language pathology is relevant to all professionals in the field, whether or not they are involved in the development of a particular curriculum. No doubt all speech-language pathologists remember some aspect of their original professional education that seemed to lack a clear rationale, or that proved frustrating in terms of how the learning experience was delivered. All practicing speech-language pathologists also will have worked at some stage alongside others whose professional preparation differed from their own, and this diversity can enrich or prove challenging in the workplace. Speech-language pathologists providing professional education experiences for students frequently will be concerned regarding the congruence or lack of congruence between their own understandings and what the students are being taught. Speech-language pathologists involved in the work of their professional association will be contributing to shared understandings regarding the knowledge and competencies required for entry to the profession, and may be involved in the accreditation processes of educational programs by the professional association. Academic staff providing speech-language pathology education will be involved in delivering curriculum to which they may or may not have had input during the development process and also may be involved in ongoing development of curriculum. Curriculum is important to all speech-language pathologists because it is the means by which the thinking and practice of future practitioners will be shaped. In all fields, not just speech-language pathology, the study of curriculum theory and the processes of curriculum development have tended to remain within the province of specialized educationalists, with many disciplinary specialists operating on the assumption that their knowledge of the field is a sufficient guide to the development of teaching. Speech-language pathologists are fortunate in having a strong theoretical background in psychological and social learning theories, and this can be seen to have influenced many of the curriculum designs and developments worldwide (see, for example, the themed issue of *Folia Phoniatrica et Logopaedica*—volume 58 in 2006). Very little has been written about the development of speech-language pathology curriculum, however, and this chapter represents an attempt to examine some of the critical issues associated with the promotion of learning and teaching in the discipline.

What Is a Curriculum?

Tanner and Tanner (2007) describe the function of educational curriculum as " . . . the systematic organization and interpretation of the culture's knowledge and skills needed for the growth of the rising generation" (p. 98). The term *curriculum* comes from Latin: The verb *currere* means "to run," as in a race, with the noun form (*curriculum*) designating variously the race itself, the race course, or a lap around the track—so the English word is well rooted in its dual sense of both product and process, occurring in real time within certain constraints with a specified end. Much of the work on curriculum has arisen in relation to education through the high school level but is equally applicable to higher education contexts. As Hewitt (2006) discusses, the cultural focus of curriculum has been present since the

days of Plato, with discussion of the ways in which to prepare young people for citizenship, whereas the focus on individual moral and cognitive development is historically more recent, associated with the work of Rousseau in the 1700s. The ideas associated with progressive education emerged in the early twentieth century through the work of such people as John Dewey (Dewey, 1916/1966), and the major social changes after the second World War were associated with movements toward greater equity in education such as that embodied in the work of Friere (1996). More recently, the study of education has been embroiled in "curriculum wars," in which critical perspectives have highlighted the ideological assumptions embodied in curriculum developments (Apple, 2004c). This ideological conflict involves the polarization of the same tensions between modern (positivist) and postmodern approaches that are discussed elsewhere in this book (see Chapter 2): At the extremes of these points of view, curriculum can be seen either as encapsulating knowledge as a "given" set of information and skills (positivist) or as a collation of socially constructed knowledge sets, each of equivalent value (postpositivist). As an alternative to these extreme positions, Moore and Young (2001) argue for a social realist perspective of knowledge, which allows for recognition of knowledge as socially and historically produced while maintaining the importance of determining relative value of knowledge for the purposes of the development of educational curriculum.

Even among those working in academic institutions, however, the notion of curriculum means different things.

In their qualitative study, Fraser and Bosanquet (2006) looked at academics' conceptions of curriculum and found four main ways of looking at this notion: first, in terms of structure and content of particular discrete units of study; second, in terms of structure and content of entire programs of study; third, in terms of students' experiences and enablement of learning; and fourth, in terms of a dynamic and interactive process of teaching and learning resulting in empowerment of students. The first two conceptions see curriculum as a product, with learning led by the teacher; the second two conceptions see curriculum as a process, with increasing contribution from learners. Fraser and Bosanquet relate these conceptions to the ideas of Habermas regarding the constituents of knowledge, whereby the notion of curriculum as product relates to the technical aspect of knowledge, the notion of curriculum as learner experience and enablement guided by the teacher relates to practical (communicative) aspects of knowledge, and the notion of curriculum as empowering relates to the emancipatory aspect of knowledge. This same distinction in relation to Habermas' perspective has been drawn in relation to professional education and its priority focus on praxis—that is, the theory of practice (rather than a separation of theory) (Grundy, 1987). As discussed later on, in speech-language pathology, as with other professional education programs, substantial external forces for curriculum maintenance and change associated with accreditation are in place. These forces render the speech-language pathology curriculum to be largely either technical or practical (in Habermas' terms)—that is, the disciplinary specifications of speech-language programs work against their capacity to be emancipatory in nature.

Beyond the documented discourse of curriculum, critical theorists have argued for the presence of a "hidden" curriculum, such that the power relationships inherent in the selection and transmission of knowledge teach students about whose voice is most powerful in society, and about how to conform to societal norms (Buras & Apple, 2006). The hidden curriculum describes the role of education in making the ideology behind what is being taught seem as if it were the only way that things in society can exist, in setting up the justification for the way things are—that is, unequal. These ideas regarding the hidden curriculum have been strongly influenced by the work of Foucault, in the recognition that the discourses that are privileged within curriculum represent the power relationships within the social order, and that education acts as a means by which such privileging of certain forms of knowledge is perpetuated. Apple (2004a) describes this status quo as being achieved through the way curriculum treats conflict as a static state. For example, teaching within science involves the exposition of the different paradigms as bodies of knowledge, and what is taught is how to come to a consensus view. Conflict as a dynamic process is not taught or, if recognized, is seen as negative (Apple, 2004a).

Tanner and Tanner (2007) incorporate this concept of hidden curriculum within their view of "collateral" curriculum, through which students learn powerful attitudinal stances to education and its applications through the combination of curricular and extracurricular learning experiences. Through the collateral curriculum, cultural reproduction is both explicitly and implicitly mediated through the processes of education. Also, Gibson (2004) discusses the "circumstantial" curriculum, which is in essence the content of the emergent learning that occurs alongside the institutionalized curriculum (e.g., learning how to interact with peer networks through meeting in the library, or the concurrent learning in part-time work unrelated to speech-language pathology). Gibson argues that these key personal and institutional ways of learning form the links between culture and individual experience that constitute the social patterns of thinking, talking, and acting that Bourdieu describes as "habitus" (Gibson, 2004).

All of these aspects of curriculum could be studied in many ways in order to explore how speech-language pathologists learn their patterns of thinking, talking, and acting, but in this chapter, the highly institutional character of the discourse of curriculum forms the main focus. All discourses are embedded within cultural institutions within society, but not always as obviously as in the case of curriculum. The main institutional contexts in which speech-language pathology curriculum is embedded involve the educational institutions, the employing institutions, and professional associations, each type of which is embedded within the government institutions from which they derive their legitimacy. According to Bernstein (1996), curriculum forms the means by which the social knowledge and values of a community are transformed into the discourse of teaching, which in turn transforms the consciousness of learners. Bernstein proposes that this process of transformation is governed by social rules associated with power relationships—for the distribution of knowledge, for how knowledge can be recontextualized for the purposes of learning, and for how learning and teaching can be evaluated.

Institutional Distribution of Knowledge through Curriculum

Education that fosters knowledge of a discipline is seen as a form of cultural capital within the work of the educationalist Bernstein and the philosopher Bourdieu, because education can be seen as a commodity in the same way as economic capital is a commodity. As with economic capital, cultural capital is distributed unequally in society, and within university institutions the value of different sorts of cultural capital is unequally distributed between disciplines (Apple, 2004b). The unequal distribution of the cultural capital of education is seen as strongly linked to social class, with Bourdieu arguing that education has as its unexamined assumption the ways of thinking and the discourse of the middle class and the assumption that all people have equal access to these discourses (Bourdieu, 1991). As noted by Bruner (1996), the notion of class and education has proved discomforting in the debates in education; this researcher suggests that the debate has been replaced by discourse about ability or intelligence in determining distribution of access to education. According to Bruner, however, in view of the impact of socioeconomic differences on developmental opportunity, the use of levels of ability as an index used by gatekeepers to education is essentially a cloak for class divisions. Also, within education, different types of learning/knowledge are stratified in the sense of being valued more or less, with different groups in society having differential access to differently valued educational experiences (Young, 1971). Just as money has no value except in the sense of the goods and services for which it may be exchanged, so too is the worth of cultural capital embedded in the system of social benefits for which it can be exchanged. This exchange value is essentially symbolic: Something—such as an academic degree—stands for a particular set of values, and the domination achieved through the symbolic exchange system has been described by Bourdieu (1977) as "symbolic violence," by which he means that people are controlled, influenced, and damaged through these self-perpetuating systems.

Speech-language pathology has been involved in a sociohistorical process of developing its social legitimacy, as exemplified through its identified scope of practice (see Chapter 1). The embedding of speech-language pathology education within the high-status institutions of universities (rather than, say, institutions providing technical education) has been part of the process by which the profession has sought to increase its perceived social value. It should not then be surprising to find that applicants to speech-language pathology programs disproportionately represent the middle class, and that speech-language pathology as a disci-

pline represents knowledge and understanding of communication disorder and difference from this privileged perspective.

Curriculum as Recontextualizing Knowledge

Tanner and Tanner (2007) describe curriculum as reconstructing cultural knowledge, in the sense that the curriculum developer reconstructs knowledge for the learner, and the learner reconstructs what is taught into personal understanding, with learning as emergent from this process. This process of reconstruction or recontextualization is highly constrained by the culture. As described by Bourdieu (1971), education sets out an intellectual map in which the learner is ostensibly free to roam, but the learner cannot go off the map itself—that is, curriculum constrains learning within cultural boundaries. Such ideas echo the early pioneering work of Dewey (1916/1966) in which he argued that education is about fostering the acquisition of the habits that allow people to fit into society (p. 46). Dewey did not view this acquisition of habits as a static conformity but instead talked about the "organic plasticity" (p. 49) involved in how the learner learns to learn (p. 45). Across the work of these philosophers and educationalists runs a common thread concerning the role of education as a means of social transmission and control, achieved through language. Bernstein (1996) suggests that the sociocultural knowledge of a community is transformed into learning in two different ways: first, through the discourse associated with the regulations governing education and, second, through the discourse associated with instruction itself.

Institutional Regulation of Education

Institutional regulation of education is achieved through discourse at governmental level, such as acts of representational bodies establishing universities, policies of distribution of funding from different levels of government, and government regulations, for example, the impact of national qualifications frameworks on education (Ensor, 2004). Institutional regulation also takes place through discourse within the institution itself (e.g., degree schedules, review processes), as well as outside the institution (e.g., state-regulated accreditation).

The regulative discourse of educational institutions has been strongly influenced by broad sociocultural ideological changes over the past two decades. Naidoo and Jamieson (2005) argue that the movement toward mass education along with increased corporatization has significant effects on the relationship between the institution and its academic professionals and students (now in a customer or consumer relationship). Although the economic discourse behind the movement is that increased competition among universities (generated through publicly available performance indicators, such as benchmarks or league tables and through differential pricing of degree packages) will result in increased efficiency and quality, Naidoo and Jamie-

son argue that the risks are loss of academic innovation (in the face of risks of losing market share) and loss of student responsibility for learning (associated with the customer role). These researchers argue that this dilemma extends Bourdieu's observations of academic capital from being a medium of exchange to an extreme view of learning as a commodity and also note that this commodification of education will differentially affect social and academic groupings. For example, strongly bounded disciplines are likely to be resistant to effects, whereas interdisciplinary studies are likely to shift with market forces, and well-established universities are likely to obtain higher market shares than those achievable by newer universities, which typically serve less socioeconomically advantaged regions or populations (Naidoo & Jamieson, 2005).

Institutional Instructional Discourse

Instructional discourse has two main aspects: first, what is taught (content) and, second, how the teaching is done (method). Although arguably methods of teaching have more far-reaching impact on learners (because they determine what is *learned*, rather than what was presented), much of the focus of educational debate generally, and within the speech-language pathology profession, tends to center on content issues (for instance, what does an entry-level speech-language pathologist need to know?). These two aspects of instructional discourse intertwine in the long-running debates regarding the relative merits of specialized, disciplinary-specific versus generic knowledge, skills, and attributes (such as critical thinking, for example), because processes of teaching play a major role in the facilitation of generic abilities. Before turning to a consideration of this debate, the following discussion examines the issues surrounding disciplinary discourse in education.

The identification of disciplinary-specific knowledges is recognized by Foucault as one of the important processes through which particular social groupings build their power base, and disciplinary-specific discourses can be seen as roughly equivalent to Kuhn's notions of paradigms (McHoul & Grace, 1993). Historically, in speech-language pathology, whether or not speech-language pathology was in fact a separate discipline was the subject of considerable debate (Siegel & Ingham, 1987); this period of debate may have marked the process of emergence as a recognized field of study, in which, as Clark (2006) argues (in relation to the emergence of computing as a discipline), the initial close association with other high-status recognized fields was disengaged through the recognition of the specificity of applications. The strong disciplinary focus of speech-language pathology education mirrors the unidisciplinary approach in much of service delivery (see Chapter 5), and just as debates about interdisciplinary practice can be seen to reflect power struggles, so too are the debates concerning moves toward interdisciplinary education (as in generic health professional programs). The experience of interdisciplinary studies, such as gender studies in the 1970s and 1980s, has been that in terms of power within the institution, such interdisciplinary

programs are effectively marginalized, largely as a result of their nonalignment with organizational structures (which remain disciplinary-based) (Bird, 2001; Burghardt & Colbeck, 2005). Speech-language pathology programs generally are found to be organizationally nested within strong disciplinary organizational structures (e.g., medicine or education faculties), fighting for recognition as allied yet separate, and frequently speaking the rhetoric of interdisciplinarity yet fundamentally concerned to retain disciplinary control.

Across all curricula, not just speech-language pathology, generic abilities are seen as important outcomes of education through which governments can monitor the effectiveness of institutions, disciplines, and programs, and such outcome measures often are linked to funding within and across institutions and thus reflect the ideological issues associated with corporatization outlined in the previous section. In his phenomenographic study exploring how academic professionals across a range of disciplines understand the construct of generic attributes of graduates of educational programs, Barrie (2006) noted the essential interchangeability of the terms "generic," "key," and "core" and of the terms "attributes," "competencies," and "skills," (any of which might include "attitudes"). Barrie identified a hierarchy of constructs regarding graduate attributes: precursory (what students bring to learning, before adding disciplinary learning), complementary (alongside disciplinary learning), translatory (generalizing disciplinary learning), and enabling (means whereby disciplinary learning is accomplished). This hierarchy ranks these understandings along a continuum of lower to higher integration with disciplinary learning, and the higher conceptions subsume the lower (and the lower preclude the higher).

For speech-language pathology, both generic and discipline-specific skills contribute to the employability of graduates, whereas for less specialized programs, the constructs of generic attributes constitute a major contributing factor determining employability (Cox & King, 2006). Knight and Yorke (2002) emphasize the importance of employability: The economic success of a society has come to be strongly associated with the education of its workforce—that is, the development of the human capital of a society is considered to result in economic growth and development.

Both generic and disciplinary attributes are sought by accrediting bodies, and by employing institutions. For example, in speech-language pathology in Australia, the professional association developed the statement of competencies for entry-level practitioners (*Competency based occupational standards for speech pathologists—entry level (revised)*, 2001) that is used in the accreditation process, and this association also was a partner in the development of the educational assessment tool for evaluating students' generic and professional competencies (S. McAllister, Lincoln, Ferguson, & McAllister, 2006). Competency-based approaches, whether generic or disciplinary-specific, can be critiqued as promoting a reductionist approach, particularly when competence is seen as an all-or-none phenomenon (Talbot, 2004). Competency approaches within Australia were driven largely through government imperatives associated with the implementation of a national qualifications framework and the need to develop a framework allowing for a process of recognizing the skills of overseas-trained immigrant workers. In the government-sponsored documents promoting this approach, however, competence in relation to higher education was argued to be necessarily a holistic notion for which indicators that captured the complexities of practice were needed (Hager & Gillis, 1995).

One of the problems with the notion of employability is that educators and employers do not necessarily share the same ideas regarding what needs to be taught. Hamilton (2005) argues that one of the challenges faced by new graduates in nursing is that they move from the educational institution in which they have demonstrated competence to the employing institution in which they are novices who are perceived as less than competent in the ways of the employed workforce. Using a foucauldian framework, Hamilton qualitatively compared the discourse of five health organizations through their written texts that were relevant for new graduates (job descriptions, performance appraisal tools, programs for new graduate employees) and texts from the undergraduate (professional qualification) curricula of seven educational institutions. The differences in how the discourses of the educating and employing institutions constructed the identity of the new graduate are summarized in Figure 8–1.

Hamilton's findings point to a major conflict between the new graduate identity as an independent knower, thinker, and decision-maker (as constructed through the discourse of knowing and thinking in education) and the new graduate identity as a part

Discourse	Theme	Educating organizations	Employing organizations
Discourse of practice	Values	• Ethical principles • Leadership, advocacy	• Ethical practices • Commitment to values of organization
	Accommodation	• Working collaboratively • Flexibility	• Working in interdisciplinary teams • Conformity and cooperation in the workplace
	Self-evaluation	• Continuous critical self-evaluation • Lifelong learning	• Participation in performance appraisal • Continuous personal and professional development
Discourse of knowing and thinking		• Independent critical and logical thinking as basis for decision-making	• Use of sound clinical reasoning
Discourse of statutes and regulation		• Meeting legal requirements	• Observing legal requirements
Discourse of the organization		• Policies and procedures for enrollment and compliance with teaching and assessment processes	• Position in relation to organizational hierarchy • Policies and procedures • Commitment to values and philosophy of organization • Promoting quality, safety, and efficiency

Drawn from the findings reported by Hamilton, H. (2005). New graduate identity: Discursive mismatch. *Contemporary Nurse, 20,* 67-77.

Figure 8–1. Comparison of the discourses within educating and employing organizations.

of the organizational structure and processes (as constructed through the bureaucratic discourse in the employing organization). Hamilton (2005) suggests that new graduates can experience dissonance in their perceived competence between these identities, and that awareness of the cultural assumptions and ideologies revealed by these discourses can inform the development of ways to assist the transition from one institution to the other. In the field of speech-language pathology, Brumfitt and colleagues looked at the transition to work, through the use of interview and focus group methods to canvass the opinions of 13 speech-language pathology managers and 31 newly graduated speech-language pathologists in one region of the United Kingdom (Brumfitt, Enderby, & Hoben, 2005). Their findings indicated the power of student clinical experiences (particularly block placements) in providing experience and expertise in real-world demands and highlighted the difficulties faced by new graduates in managing the wider administrative roles and tasks required in the workplace. Lincoln and colleagues' research provides a way forward in assisting with such transition difficulties (Lincoln, Adamson, & Cant, 2001). These researchers surveyed the perceptions of 47 experienced speech pathologists as to the managerial skills required of new graduates and found that these related to three main domains described as management of future planning (e.g., time management, planning goals for work team), organizational practices (e.g., advocacy for the work unit), and regulative knowledge and practices. Lincoln and colleagues suggest that both educational and employing

institutions have a responsibility to assist the transition of the new graduate in developing these skills. Part of this responsibility is about clinical education (see Chapter 7) and the need for authentic learning experiences in the process of instruction.

Many processes of instruction are involved in the delivery of curriculum content and are linked to power in the sense that different processes are associated with different balances of power between educators and learners. Bourdieu and Passeron (1994) discuss an empirical study of lecturers' and students' perspectives on this balance of power, which found that for both groups, the power shift in tutorial-style round table discussions are valued but perceived as challenging (for both educators and learners), whereas more formal lectures generally are more valued and less challenging to both the power of the educator and the identity of the learner. A strong argument can be made for the need to align the process of education with content objectives, because just as a hidden curriculum can be identified in the selection of content, the process of teaching reveals a hidden curriculum regarding the relationship between those in power (those who "know") and others. Learning about this relationship is especially important in speech-language pathology, with its agenda of teaching students about the process of learning for clients. So, for example, teaching client-centered therapies in a lecturer-driven curriculum sends a double message to students. If students are taught in ways that disempower them, it should not be surprising that they do therapy in ways that disempower clients. Certainly, one of the most pervasive features of the content of speech-language pathology education is the extent to which curriculum is driven by educators (working in both educating and employing institutions) and the professional association in the context of governmental constraints, and how little of the content or process is open to input by the learners. One of the most striking anomalies arises in the educational objective of developing the lifelong learning skill of *self-directed learning*, yet opportunities to choose and direct learning are rare to nonexistent within most speech-language pathology programs. Although this limitation may arise from the highly specialized nature of the disciplinary coverage, it also is increasingly apparent that because curriculum cannot keep pace with the expansion of knowledge, then the instructional task must become one of teaching students how to learn. The instructional method shapes attitudes to learning, including motivation to learn, curiosity, being comfortable with not knowing, and ability to learn in different ways, so a curriculum that empowers students to learn in diverse ways becomes essential (Cherry, 2005)

A good example of the importance of instructional process over content arises in the consideration of the teaching of multicultural awareness (see Chapter 5). From the findings of a national survey of 228 programs in the United States, Stewart and Gonzales conclude that although today's academic programs generally incorporate teaching about cultural diversity, students' clinical experiences vary greatly in the extent to which they offer direct learning opportunities for students to increase their multicultural awareness (Stewart & Gonzalez, 2002). In a recent

discussion paper, Stockman and colleagues argue that academic and clinical curriculum in speech-language pathology in the United States is not yet showing any significant progress toward achieving the professional association's goal of multicultural "infusion" (Stockman, Boult, & Robinson, 2004). Instead, academic curriculum is following a pattern of "inclusion," through identifying particular points in the curriculum at which multicultural awareness is taught as a discrete content area. The notion of "infusion" captures the recognition that learning needs to be intercultural, rather than multicultural. For example, it is not possible to teach about every different cultural group with which students may work, but it is possible to develop teaching strategies that promote intercultural skills to enable the learner to approach the "other" with curiosity (not fear), openness to a view of the world from another perspective, and the ability to communicate in this situation (Lee, 2005). These teaching strategies are built on a critical discourse perspective, enabling students to recognize and engage with diversity. Kymlicka (2003) argues that education is fundamental to building intercultural citizenship within multicultural communities, and that without intercultural awareness, multicultural communities remain politically and socially divided. As part of facilitating students' intercultural awareness, the teaching of intercultural skills demands that educators model these practices. For example, Main and colleagues distill from a larger ethnographic study some of the teaching strategies that are well suited to students from an Australian Aboriginal and Torres Strait Islander background, and these strategies (e.g., peer and collaborative teaching making use of facilitation rather than direct elicitation) are well designed for inclusivity and the modeling of intercultural communication (Main, Nichol, & Fennell, 2000).

Previously (in Chapter 6), the impact of technological developments facilitating online learning has been argued to open a bridge to academic discourses through the range of dialogic interaction available. As indicated by a survey by Tastle, White, and Shackleton (2005), the use of online learning as one of the processes of instruction is increasing, mostly offered as a way to add value to traditional modes of delivery. These researchers found that although academic professionals indicated that more time was required for preparation of this mode of delivery, the academics' perception was that only slightly better learning outcomes were obtained. McLoughlin (2001), however, argues that online delivery has a capacity for flexibility that increases the capacity for delivery of interculturally appropriate methods of education, because online learning is expanding the international delivery of higher education, thereby driving increasingly culturally diverse virtual classrooms. McLoughlin suggests that this confers advantages for all learners because intercultural skills increase employability, and online delivery allows for multiple options in how material is delivered, providing students with more choices in how to learn.

Problem-based learning is one of the methods of instruction that has been strongly promoted as allowing for considerable student self-direction, and providing for close alignment between the instructional method with the objectives of both the educating and the employing institutions, and is becoming more prominent in speech-language pathology education (M. L. Rose, 2005). Similar clashes between the educating and employing discourses, however, can be seen to arise: Feedback from medical students from a problem-based learning program moving into clinical learning indicated the need to shift their learning style from the reasoning-dominant approach required in the problem-based learning classroom to what could be described as a pattern identification model of decision-making in the clinic—in other words, these students found problems in relating theory to practice that were similar to problems encountered by students from other programs (Prince, Boshuizen, Van der Vleuten, & Scherpbier, 2005).

Across all programs in speech-language pathology, the process of teaching involves the provision of learning opportunities that attempt to facilitate this transition from theory to practice, and considerable debate is ongoing regarding the extent to which such learning experiences need to be authentic in terms of both the skills involved and the context of teaching (that is, classroom or clinic) (Brown, Collins, & Duguid, 1989). As previously noted (in Chapter 7), Cruice (2005) suggests a continuum of authenticity—for example, the use of actors in simulations (Edwards, Franke, & McGuiness, 1995), interactive video technology, and so on. In general, the input of people with communication disorders into the education curriculum content has been nearly nonexistent (except as "objects" of study, as opposed to participants), and although their role in relation to educative processes has been significant (through their willingness to participate in assessment and therapy sessions conducted by students), their involvement has been in the role of client. One of the most exciting developments in recent years has been a move to shift the social positioning of people with communication disorders from that of client to that of educator—for example in a role of "client tutor" for small group learning within a speech-language pathology education program (Beecham, 2005), reflecting a movement associated with the recognition of their status of experts in the lived experience of their disability (see Chapter 4).

The provision of in-house learning experiences allows academic institutions to maintain control over curriculum, in terms of control of content and process, as well as in terms of economic control (McKenna & Wellard, 2004), and although innovations in instructional process are couched in terms of improved educational outcomes, it is important to clearly acknowledge economic imperatives (L. McAllister, 2005; M. L. Rose, 2005). When costs of professional education become a ball to be tossed between educating and employing institutions, the quality of the education process is at risk. So, for example, in a small-scale qualitative research study of nursing students on practicum in a hospital setting, McLeland and Williams (2002) describe a situation frequently experienced among practicing speech-language pathologists. Although the students' experiences were positive overall, the reported negative experiences arose from time pressures, seen as driving a wedge between the students' rights to learning and the nurse-

educators' needs to deliver prompt, safe care: As time pressures increased, the students would be increasingly directed to specific tasks, rather than facilitated toward independent decision-making regarding holistic care, and with diminished time for reflection on practice. These researchers note that if the educator is oppressed, then so too will the student be oppressed—that is, power and powerlessness work their way down the hierarchy.

In order to provide authentic learning opportunities for speech-language pathology students, the immediacy of problems with finding placements obscures the wider issue regarding the societal value of competent speech-language practice, and the broader ideological discourses that shape how, when, and why support is provided for curriculum.

Institutional Evaluation of Curriculum

Of interest, the extent of student learning is rarely used as an index of efficacy of curriculum (as discussed further in relation to evidence-based practice in education later in the chapter). Instead, methods of student assessment constitute one index by which curriculum content and delivery can be evaluated. With regard to this approach to evaluation, the focus of evaluation involves the extent to which alignment is achieved between the curriculum objectives, the processes of delivery, and how student learning is assessed. For example, Anijar (2004) notes the increasing popularity of portfolio-based assessment, which arises from a narrative tradition of learning, yet students' portfolios typically are assessed using behaviorally identified objectives, which are essentially residue from positivist traditions of assessment. When assessment methods are out of alignment with curriculum objectives, then the educative process can be undermined. For example, Knight and Yorke (2002) argue that formative assessment methods assist in the development of self-efficacy (an attitude associated with high employability), in contrast with summative assessment methods, which tend to promote a non-risk-taking approach to learning.

Robley and colleagues present a systematic mapping process that was used to evaluate the extent to which a medical program was achieving its generic skills outcome objectives (Robley, Whittle, & Murdoch-Eaton, 2005). Using triangulation of data from documentation of student assessment tasks, interviews with students, educators from academic and clinical environments, the curriculum evaluation process involved a detailed process of mapping generic skill outcomes "delivered, declared, and learned" against objectives, and when misalignment was identified, these findings provided directions for change.

Such mapping processes are used by professional associations in their accreditation of speech-language pathology programs, although different constructs of the profession's role in evaluating curriculum make for widely divergent aspects of curriculum which are considered. So, for example, a large part of the accreditation focus for the American Speech-Language-Hearing Association (ASHA) involves the identification and evaluation of the sufficiency of resources (human and economic) for the support of the educational curriculum, and the evaluation of indices of curriculum content and processes in terms of hours of input and experience. By contrast, the focus of the accreditation process for Speech Pathology Australia is the adequacy of the processes of student assessment to determine the competence of students, in relation to the occupational standards of the profession, so this accreditation process involves mapping assessment items against competencies, rather than inputs.

As well as professional evaluation, speech-language pathology curricula are reviewed through the institutional processes required by the particular university in which they are situated. Such reviews commonly involve seeking feedback from a wide range of internal and external sources, generally including the professional association, members of the profession involved with the program, students in the program (e.g., through student satisfaction questionnaires), and employers of graduates from the program, and ideally, also incorporating input from recipients of services delivered by students and graduates from the program. The value placed on feedback from these sources as stakeholders reflects the consumerism ideology currently influencing social institutions in Western culture, as previously discussed. Although such review processes make use of quantitative data (such as that used for quality assurance and benchmarking), the review process itself commonly uses a highly interpretive methodology, making use of interviews and examination of narrative accounts in order to make recommendations, usually constrained within an institutionally imposed set of terms of reference.

Although such comprehensive reviews typically are undertaken only in 3- to 5-year cycles, routine use of indices of quality applied for benchmarking purposes across the institution, such as student enrollment and attrition rates, is increasing. To date, speech-language pathology programs rarely publish accounts of their evaluation of curriculum, and comparative benchmarking remains in its infancy. One group of investigators, however, recently embarked on a program of research moving in this direction (Lincoln, McAllister, Ferguson, & McAllister, 2006/2007).

The extent to which such evaluative processes actually shape change in curriculum is underexplored in general, and unexplored in speech-language pathology, and the forces for maintenance and change are examined in the next section.

Institutional Forces for Maintaining and Changing Curriculum

In view of common concerns among speech-language pathology academics across institutions, one of the relevant agents that would be expected to be a powerful force for curriculum change is the academic community of scholars. Paradoxically, however, this may in fact be one of the weakest forces for curriculum change—especially because no institutionalized system of peer review or other process is in place that would prompt individual educators in either academic or professional environments to respond to shifts in theory.

Even if such peer review processes were in place, the question of conflict of interest would arise, because peer academic educators often are competitors (for employment positions or research grants, for example). Thus, although large shifts in professional practice have an institutional mechanism for influencing curriculum (accreditation), theoretical paradigmatic shifts may be idiosyncratically adopted across different programs, as found in the uptake of new phonological theories (Nelson & Ball, 2003). When the professional association's process of accreditation is silent, then considerable diversity emerges in both theory and practice as taught through curriculum. For example, Yaruss and Quesal (2002) looked at the inclusion of stuttering within curriculum across 159 ASHA-accredited programs. These investigators found that only half included coursework in fluency and that two thirds of the programs did not provide practicum experience in stuttering. These investigators associated this diminution of curriculum coverage of stuttering with the change to the ASHA accreditation framework in 1993, which moved from the previously required 25 hours of clinical practicum in fluency to fluency experience's being subsumed within requirement for practicum in "speech" (Yaruss & Quesal, 2002).

Although external social forces work to change curriculum, internal forces may work to maintain it. Arnold (2004) argues that internal curricular reform inevitably involves a political dimension, such that although a reform may proceed on rationalist grounds, the political nature of institutions will shape the outcome. Arnold presents a case study of a university in which a process of curricular reform of under-graduate studies resulted in fact in very little actual change, largely owing to the territorial defense of the organizational disciplinary structures. In fact, the only real change observed in the study was that the recognition of the need for compliance with requirements for cultural diversity education was met with the inclusion of a required course on the subject (see comments on intercultural curriculum earlier in this chapter). Arnold argues, however, that what did take place was "symbolic action," in the sense of explicitly reviewing the mission of the institution against the objectives of the members of the institution, and that such symbolic action was still worthwhile in sociopolitical terms of increasing the organization's prestige (as an institution open to review) and attracting resources (a mechanism for which was attached to the review process). Arnold does not hold this view as a cynical position, but it must be asked whether the examination of the institutional symbolic system in this situation was one of shoring up social positioning, rather than one of critical examination, because no real symbolic action occurred other than a reiteration of alignments.

Bernstein, writing in the early 1970s, identified two broad approaches to curriculum structure: closed and open (Bernstein, 1971). The *closed* structure was associated with collections of knowledge, such as disciplinary modules, with a teacher-led vertical hierarchy in its administration and development, and was seen to be relatively impermeable to societal influences. The *open* structure was associated with integration of knowledges across disciplines and student direction in terms of

learning foci and methods and was seen to be highly responsive to societal influences. Of interest, Bernstein did not categorize either approach as being of more or less value; instead, he queried whether movements toward open models of education could be "symptoms of moral crisis" (Bernstein, 1996, p. 67), which, rather than being an end in themselves, constitute a stage toward change and development of more stable forms of curriculum.

This notion is echoed in the discussion by Pillay, Kathard, and Samuel (1997) of a curriculum framework for speech-language pathology and audiology in the context of the post-apartheid reforms in South Africa. These investigators argue that the empirical-analytical paradigms that have predominated in speech-language pathology have separated theory and practice, placing them in a hierarchical relationship, which is "framed-in" (Pillay et al., p. 115) and unsuited to the challenges of the need to make changes in practice. Instead, they argue, a critical paradigm involves reflexivity between theory and practice and emancipatory goals for learners and thus " . . . promotes the curriculum as a *dynamic entity*—such as that associated with the dynamism of social transformation" (Pillay et al., p. 115). Bernstein (1996), however, does note that more integrated (open) educational discourse may work productively toward creating social order in situations characterized by a high degree of ideological consensus among academic staff (and presumably among learners). Speech-language pathology curriculum, as has previously been discussed, tends toward a more closed curriculum state in terms of relatively stable disciplinary boundaries and structure, but possibly because of the close relationship between these programs and the profession, both operating within the same community of practice, considerable opportunity exists for ordered responsivity in curriculum development. As Bernstein (1971) says, the nineteenth century demanded an education system that promoted people to be "submissive and inflexible," but the demands of the twenty-first century are for an education system that fosters people who are "conforming but flexible" (p. 67).

Expert Practice and Curriculum: The Example of Evidence-Based Practice

Evidence-based policy and practice have emerged only since the early 1990s but have rapidly become a pervasive influence across health and education (see also Chapter 2). In view of the nature of curriculum as essentially conforming (Cope, 2005), the advent of this movement and its influence on curriculum provides an illustrative case study of the interrelationship between expert practice and curriculum. Evidence-based practice " ... is the integration of best research evidence with clinical expertise and patient values" (Sackett, Straus, Richardson, Rosenberg, & Haynes, 2000, p. 1), but much of the focus on evidence-based practice has been on what constitutes "best" research and what constitutes "evidence" (Drake, Latimer, Leff, McHugo, & Burns, 2004; Stiwne & Dahlgren, 2004), rather than on how it

is integrated with either clinical expertise or patient values. The issues for curriculum development in regard to evidence based practice thus rests not only on the learning and teaching related to the nature of "best" research, and to the nature of "evidence," but also on the development of the expertise needed to integrate these understandings with practice, and on the development of awareness of the role of patient values in the process.

The expertise involved in evidence-based practice is in part institutionalized through the development of guidelines for practice as a bridge between the research and the practitioner. Such guidelines are drawn up by expert panels (Reilly, Oates, & Douglas, 2004) comprising experts in critical appraisal, experts in practice, and user groups (patients, self-help groups; refer to Chapter 4 regarding the role of advocacy). With reference to speech-language pathology, Reilly and colleagues dismiss concerns regarding the potential for political interference and concerns that guidelines arising out of evidence-based practice will erode professional autonomy (Reilly, Oates, et al., p. 320) and call on institutions (professional associations, universities, and employers) to work toward the development of evidence-based guidelines for practice. Tellingly, the professional association that has produced the greatest number of guidelines—the Royal College for Speech Language Therapists— has done so within the context of a wide-scale government initiative across the health sector; this correlation underscores the strong political climate driving the development of such guidelines. In the field of mental health, Tanenbaum (2003) explicitly notes that, despite the theoretical and practical concerns surrounding evidence-based practice, the push toward greater use of evidence based practice serves the important political purpose of increasing public awareness of appropriate interventions and directing government funding initiatives to worthwhile services.

According to Colyer and Kamath (1999), the expert clinician also is seen as the one who is making judgments about how and when to apply the external clinical evidence (evidence-based research) to the clinical evidence derived from the interaction with the patient (case history, physical examination, test results and so on. The equal importance of clinical expertise and of the external evidence base is well expressed by these investigators: "Without clinical expertise, practice may become tyrannized by evidence that is inapplicable or inappropriate for an individual patient. Without best evidence, practice runs the risk of becoming both ineffective and inefficient" (Colyer & Kamath, p. 189).

The "best" evidence is an ideologically derived determination, and although much of the debate tends to center on qualitative versus quantitative paradigms, if not all research is equally "good" even within ideological paradigms, then the question still remains of how to evaluate research within or across paradigms. Forbes and colleagues (1999) note that researchers from widely divergent ideological perspectives (influenced by postpositivism, interpretism, critical social theory, and feminism) all still need to think about this notion of "best" research. According to these investigators, what professionals working from these divergent

perspectives have in common in their search for best research is the close examination and critical analysis of methodological rigor by the community of scholars and practitioners, the examination of the methods by which observations and interpretations are corroborated, and the presence of sufficient scope to address the questions or problems under study.

Such contesting paradigms of research are not the sole ideological influence on evidence-based practice. Evidence-based practice itself can be seen as embedded within what Colyer and Kamath (1999) describe as the dominant liberal ideology (promoting values of individual freedom, choice, and responsibility within a strong capitalist society), which has moved health care services to be seen from the view of the market place and consumerism. This ideology has resulted in a focus on clinical effectiveness and efficiency, and evidence-based practice is part of that focus. This ideology thus has two inbuilt contesting discourses: that of quality and best practice, competing with that of economic efficiency (that is, quality limited to that deliverable within available resources); see Figure 8–2.

Evidence-Based Practice in Speech-Language Pathology

In 1995, Enderby and Emerson suggested that not all subspecialties within speech-language pathology were equally influenced by movement toward efficacy research (Enderby & Emerson, 1995), with those subspecialties that were tied more closely to medicine and thus more closely linked to the scientific paradigm showing the greater

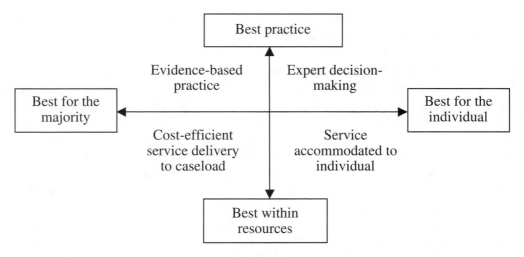

Figure 8–2. Competing discourses in evidence-based policy and practice.

influence. By 2004, the work of Reilly and colleagues indicated that although considerable diversity was still present in the types of research contributing to the evidence base across subspecialties within speech-language pathology, evidence-based practice was widespread across the discipline (Reilly, Douglas, & Oates, 2004).

Although evidence-based practice may be talked about in the profession, application is less than ideal in the workplace (Reilly, Oates, et al., 2004). The barriers to the transfer from evidence to practice are discussed in terms of problems of individual practitioners, such as traditions of trial-and-error problem-solving or limitations associated with learning styles (M. Rose & Baldac, 2004, p. 319), and problems accessing the research literature (both practically and in terms of understanding the research genre) (Reilly, Oates, et al., 2004, p. 336), or in terms of individual dissatisfaction or dissonance with the ideology perspective of evidence-based practice. In contrast, Mykhalovskiy and Weir (2004) argue that critiques of evidence-based practice need to widen beyond focusing solely on concerns regarding covert agendas for rationalization of services and concerns for the loss of the patient's perspective (as discussed later). Instead, these investigators argue, the transfer of evidence to practice is in itself worth problematizing[1] because of the gulf between the highly empirical-rationalist discourse associated with the best research and its application through highly interpretive expert clinical reasoning processes. Arguably, the problems with transfer of evidence to practice are more fundamentally related to issues arising from these issues to do with both this dissonance between the expert

---

[1]The term 'problematize' is used within a critical perspective to describe the process of standing back from the typical way in which issue is described or understood in order to study how the description or understanding itself has emerged from its social context, and how the description or understanding is maintained within the social context of the problem.

decision-making processes and the nature of evidences (from the research and as observed in the patient).

As a case example, the report by Packman and colleagues (2003) of diverse and inconsistent application of an evidence-based stuttering intervention was discussed by Reilly, Oates and Douglas (2004) as exemplifying barriers to evidence-based practice. This example also highlights the problem inherent in application of evidence to practice through expert clinical reasoning. A majority of the barriers listed were essentially institutional—for example, workplace restrictions on number of sessions that could be offered, or what sort of timing (block or weekly). Although these problems were seen as resting with individual professionals not communicating with managers, a more likely explanation involves a broader view in which discourses of economics are competing with the "best practice" discourse of evidence-based practice (see Figure 8–2). If these competing discourses are not recognized, the individual practitioner is left arguing "best practice" in the face of calls for "better research." The practitioner is shadow-boxing, trying to fight a battle for evidence-based services in a context within which the "best" is never good enough, because this is not the actual basis for institutional decision-making (see also discussion of these issues in Chapter 4).

Curriculum and Evidence-Based Practice

In making recommendations for the teaching of evidence-based practice, Sackett and colleagues (2000) argue that it is not enough to teach critical analysis and appraisal skills, because in order for learners (whether students or graduates undertaking professional development) to apply evidence, the method of teaching needs to be both patient-centered (that is, with a focus on cases and case management decision-making) and learner-centered (that is, adjusted for what the learner is ready and able to take on board in the particular context of teaching, whether that be in the classroom or on the run in a ward situation). The largest shift in teaching urged by Sackett and colleagues is that in order for the learner to develop the skills to identify, evaluate, and apply evidence, the teacher needs to relinquish the role of "knower" and become an active co-participant in the learning process, enabling both modeling of the decision-making processes involved and emergent learning for the student. Rose and Baldac (2004) argue that problem-based learning is an ideal alignment of teaching methodology with the objectives of teaching how to apply evidence to practice situations (pp. 326–327). Whether problem-based learning delivery is used or not, these researchers make some useful suggestions for teaching critical application—for instance, creating learning environments in which learners discover both availability and lack of available evidence, and in which learners can explore diverse perspectives and have opportunities to challenge accepted practice. Rose and Baldac also note that assessment methods also need to be aligned with teaching objectives and method (as previously discussed in this chapter).

Rose and Baldac suggest that some academic educators also may be resistant to evidence-based practice (Rose & Baldac, 2004, p. 327) and hence resistant to incorporating this approach within the curriculum (and perhaps tending to "include" rather than "infuse" the curriculum). Again, these investigators suggest such resistance to be individualized as resistance to change, or as the need for additional time for preparation. It must be recognized, however, that evidence-based practice has not been conclusively shown to improve practice or outcomes for clients (Colyer & Kamath, 1999)—so the educator faces a decision regarding the extent to which this movement is in effect a reframing of perspectives, and the extent to which this should influence the curriculum. In view of the conforming nature of curriculum in general, institutional influences, both external and internal, can be expected to render different curricula more or less responsive to evidence-based practice. As Griffiths (2005) points out, however, in critiquing or resisting evidence-based practice, the risk is that the reverse situation may be fostered, wherein poor practice is defended. Instead, Griffiths suggests, part of teaching evidence-based practice also is about raising learners' awareness of evidence-based practice as a genre, with its own rules for what are the elements of value within it (that is, measurable outcomes, rather than interpersonal processes) and their interrelationship, so that learners can deconstruct it and use it knowingly (Freshwater, 2004).

Ethical Issues and Evidence-Based Practice

The critique of evidence-based practice from a humanist perspective argues that evidence-based practice " . . . strips patients of their stories and the meaning of their experience, reducing them to passive recipients of doctor-centered communications" (Mykhalovskiy & Weir, 2004, p. 1062). Colyer and Kamath (1999) point out that the implicit ethical base for evidence-based practice is utilitarian, that is, the greatest good for the greatest number; thus, a particular treatment approach is of value if effective for most if not for all individuals. As these investigators note, clinicians' expert decision-making processes are applied within individual relationships, which entails ethical decision-making within that interrelationship—thereby presenting yet another conflict. Maseide (2006) tackles this issue, noting that the clinician considers multiple lines of evidence in any given situation, including the evidence observed in the physical state of the patient, the evidence arising out of tests and documented reports on the patient, and the discourse about the patient that occurs in discussions in case conferences, as well as the published scientific evidence. Maseide states that " . . . evidence is essential, but its meaning and use is often grounded in moral and situational considerations rather than in scripts based on general scientific and evidence-based guidelines or principles of administrative governance" (p. 53). Maseide examined the clinical decision-making in a cancer ward, noting the contribution of such factors as patients' age or apparent "courage" (for example) to shaping discussions and decision-making, along with the platform of scientific evidence. Thus at a local, patient-by-patient level, ethics and science mingle discursively.

At the more global level of service provision, although evidence-based practice argues for a role for expert clinical decision-making and patient rights, two competing discourses are in use—one promoting the individual patient's rights to best practice and choice, and the other promoting the needs for services to be considered collectively for the community as a whole, in terms of greatest benefit for the majority. These competing discourses (summarized in Figure 8–2) present important professional and ethical challenges for clinicians. In discussing similar issues for mental health nursing, Lines (2001) argues that deconstruction of these competing discourses enables the break away from the artificial polarization of these viewpoints, instead enabling a movement toward an understanding of how different discourses arise and why. From a critical discourse perspective, the aim is to recognize, and make evident, the competing discourses as the foundation for working through the decision-making required for service delivery and patient care.

Evidence-Based Curriculum

As previously indicated, the field of education has been slow to pick up the influence of evidence-based policy and practice, perhaps because of the very different ideological discourses within the field (which tend to be interpretive, rather than empirical-analytical). Questions regarding efficacy, however, are important to explore in attempting to develop curriculum: For example, what curriculum suits individual learners, or most of them? What curriculum serves the community in general or vested interests in the community? What is

the "best" education ? What is the best education that can be delivered within the resources available?

Oakley (2006) discusses the resistance of academics to the application of systematic reviews and randomized controlled trials as associated with evidence-based policy and practice in the field of education. She analyzed four "resistance" texts that articulated views opposing the use of these methodologies in evaluation of education and identified the main themes expressed as involving rejection of the positivist paradigm on ideological grounds (from postmodern perspective) and on practical grounds (difficulties with feasibility), as well as on political grounds (as tools of government control). Oakley then presents a summary of the systematic reviews and randomized controlled trials in education (e.g., from the Cochrane Library) and uses these data to underscore the practicality of the methodology and to point out instances in which results have in fact contradicted government policy directions. A majority of systematic reviews in education have placed high weight on the evidence from qualitative studies; according to Oakley, this may represent a movement within the evidence-based paradigm toward greater integration of interpretive perspectives, so these methodologies should be seen as tools, rather than as ideological threats.

Concluding Comments

This chapter has explored the role of the diverse discourses associated with curriculum for speech-language pathology, with an emphasis on the institutional character of curriculum. Curriculum has been argued to be the fundamental tool for cultural reproduction of the discipline, but the institutions in which curriculum is embedded are themselves products of the culture in which they occur.

References

Anijar, K. (2004). (Open peer commentaries) Discourse as rock formation: Fruitcake as professionalism. *American Journal of Bioethics*, 4(2), W8–W10.

Apple, M. W. (2004a). The hidden curriculum and the nature of conflict. In *Ideology and curriculum* (3rd ed., pp. 77–97). New York: Routledge.

Apple, M. W. (2004b). Ideology and cultural and economic reproduction. In *Ideology and curriculum* (3rd ed., pp. 25–40). New York: Routledge.

Apple, M. W. (2004c). *Ideology and curriculum* (3rd ed.). New York: Routledge.

Arnold, G. B. (2004). Symbolic politics and institutional boundaries in curriculum reform: The case of national sectarian university. *Journal of Higher Education*, 75(5), 572–593.

Barrie, S. C. (2006). Understanding what we mean by the generic attributes of graduates. *Higher Education*, 51, 215–241.

Beecham, R. (2005). "Clients" as teachers: Power-sharing in the speech-language therapy curriculum. *Advances in Speech-Language Pathology*, 7(3), 130–137.

Bernstein, B. (1971). On the classification and framing of educational knowledge. In M. F. D. Young (Ed.), *Knowledge and control: New directions for the sociology of education* (chap. 2, pp. 47–69). London: Collier-Macmillan.

Bernstein, B. (1996). *Pedagogy, symbolic control, and identity: Theory, research, critique*. London: Taylor & Francis.

Bird, E. (2001). Disciplining the interdisciplinary: Radicalism and the academic curriculum. *British Journal of Sociology of Education*, 22(4), 463–478.

Bourdieu, P. (1971). Systems of education and systems of thought. In M. F. D. Young (Ed.), *Knowledge and social control: New directions for the sociology of education* (chap. 2, pp. 189–207). London: Collier-Macmillan.

Bourdieu, P. (1977). *Outline of a theory of practice* (R. Nice, Trans.). Cambridge, NY: Cambridge University Press.

Bourdieu, P. (1991). *Language and symbolic power* (G. Raymond & M. Adamson, Trans.). Oxford: Polity Press.

Bourdieu, P., & Passeron, J. (1994). Introduction: Language and relationship to language in the teaching situation (R. Teese, Trans.). In P. Bourdieu, J. Passeron, & M. de Saint Martin (Eds.), *Academic discourse: Linguistic misunderstanding and professorial power* (pp. 1–34). Cambridge, UK: Polity Press.

Brown, J. S., Collins, A., & Duguid, P. (1989, Jan-Feb). Situated cognition and the culture of learning. *Educational Researcher*, 32–42.

Brumfitt, S., Enderby, P., & Hoben, K. (2005). The transition to work of newly qualified speech and language therapists: Implications for the curriculum. *Learning in Health and Social Care*, 4(3), 142–155.

Bruner, J. S. (1996). *The culture of education*. Cambridge, Mass: Harvard University Press.

Buras, K. L., & Apple, M. W. (2006). Introduction. In M. W. Apple & K. L. Buras (Eds.), *The subaltern speak: Curriculum, power, and educational struggles* (pp. 1–39). London: Routledge.

Burghardt, D. A., & Colbeck, C. L. (2005). Women's studies faculty at the intersection of institutional power and feminist values. *Journal of Higher Education*, 76(3), 301–330.

Cherry, N. L. (2005). Preparing for practice in the age of complexity. *Higher Education Research & Development*, 24(4), 309–320.

Clark, M. (2006). A case study in the acceptance of a new discipline. *Studies in Higher Education, 31*(2), 133–148.

Colyer, H., & Kamath, P. (1999). Evidence-based practice. A philosophical and political analysis: Some matters for consideration by professional practitioners. *Journal of Advanced Nursing, 29*(1), 188–193.

Competency based occupational standards for speech pathologists—entry level (revised). (2001). Melbourne: Speech Pathology Australia.

Cope, N. (2005). Apprenticeship reinvented: Cognition, discourse and implications for academic literacy. *Prospect, 20*(3), 42–62.

Cox, S., & King, D. (2006). Skill sets: An approach to embed employability in course design. *Education & Training, 48*(4), 262–274.

Cruice, M. (2005). Common issues but alternative solutions and innovations. *Advances in Speech-Language Pathology, 7*(3), 162–166.

Dewey, J. (1916/1966). *Democracy and education: An introduction to the philosophy of education.* New York: Free Press.

Drake, R. E., Latimer, E. A., Leff, H. S., McHugo, G. J., & Burns, B. J. (2004). What is evidence? *Child and Adolescent Psychiatric Clinics of North America, 13,* 717–728.

Edwards, H., Franke, M., & McGuiness, B. (1995). Using simulated patients to teach clinical reasoning. In J. Higgs & M. Jones (Eds.), *Clinical reasoning in the health professions* (pp. 269–278). Oxford: Butterworth Heinemann.

Enderby, P., & Emerson, J. (1995). *Does speech and language therapy work? A review of the literature.* London: Whurr.

Ensor, P. (2004). Contesting discourses in higher education curriculum restructuring in South Africa. *Higher Education, 48,* 339–359.

Forbes, D., King, K. M., Kushner, K. E., Letourneau, N. L., Myrick, A., Florence, A., et al. (1999). Warrantable evidence in nursing science. *Journal of Advanced Nursing, 29*(2), 373–379.

Fraser, S. P., & Bosanquet, A. M. (2006). The curriculum? That's just a unit outline, isn't it? *Studies in Higher Education, 31*(3), 269–284.

Freire, P. (1996). *Pedagogy of the oppressed* (M. Bergman Ramos, Trans.). London: Penguin.

Freshwater, D. (2004). *Deconstructing evidence-based practice.* London: Routledge.

Gibson, P. (2004). Life and learning in further education: Constructing the circumstantial curriculum. *Journal of Further and Higher Education, 28*(3), 333–346.

Griffiths, P. (2005). Evidence-based practice: A deconstruction and postmodern critique: Book review article. *International Journal of Nursing Studies, 42,* 355–361.

Grundy, S. (1987). *Curriculum: Product or praxis?* London: Falmer Press.

Hager, P., & Gillis, S. (1995). Assessment at higher levels. In W. C. Hall (Ed.), *Key aspects of competency-based assessment* (pp. 59–71). Adelaide, Australia: NCVER.

Hamilton, H. (2005). New graduate identity: Discursive mismatch. *Contemporary Nurse, 20,* 67–77.

Hewitt, T. W. (2006). *Understanding and shaping curriculum.* Thousand Oaks, CA: Sage.

Knight, P. T., & Yorke, M. (2002). Employability through curriculum. *Tertiary Education and Management, 8*(4), 261–276.

Kymlicka, W. (2003). Multicultural states and intercultural citizens. *Theory and research in education, 1*(2), 147–169.

Lee, T. M. L. (2005). Intercultural teaching in higher education. *Intercultural Education, 16*(3), 201–215.

Lincoln, M., Adamson, B. J., & Cant, R. V. (2001). The importance of managerial competencies for new graduates in speech pathology. *Advances in Speech-Language Pathology, 3*(1), 25–26.

Lincoln, M., McAllister, S., Ferguson, A., & McAllister, L. (2006/2007). *Benchmarking clinical learning in speech pathology to support assessment, discipline standards, teaching innovation and student learning.* Project funded by The Carrick Institute for

Learning and Teaching in Higher Education. Sydney: University of Sydney.

Lines, K. (2001). A philosophical analysis of evidence-based practice in mental health nursing. *Australian and New Zealand Journal of Mental Health Nursing, 10,* 167–175.

Main, D., Nichol, R., & Fennell, R. (2000). Reconciling pedagogy and health sciences to promote indigenous health. *Australian and New Zealand Journal of Public Health, 24*(2), 211–213.

Maseide, P. (2006). The deep play of medicine: Discursive and collaborative processing of evidence in medical problem solving. *Communication & Medicine, 3*(1), 43–54.

McAllister, L. (2005). Issues and innovations in clinical education. *Advances in Speech-Language Pathology, 7*(3), 138–148.

McAllister, S., Lincoln, M., Ferguson, A., & McAllister, L. (2006). *COMPASS™ (competency assessment in speech pathology) assessment and resource manual.* Melbourne: Speech Pathology Australia.

McHoul, A., & Grace, W. (1993). *A Foucault primer: Discourse, power and the subject.* Melbourne: Melbourne University Press.

McKenna, L. G., & Wellard, S. J. (2004). Discursive influences on clinical teaching in Australian undergraduate nursing program. *Nurse Education Today, 24,* 229–235.

McLeland, A., & Williams, A. (2002). An emancipatory praxis study of nursing students on clinical practicum in New Zealand: Pushed to the peripheries. *Contemporary Nurse, 12,* 185–193.

McLoughlin, C. (2001). Inclusivity and alignment: Principles of pedagogy, task and assessment design for effective cross-cultural online learning. *Distance Education, 22*(1), 7–29.

Moore, R., & Young, M. (2001). Knowledge and the curriculum in the sociology of education: Towards a reconceptualisation. *British Journal of Sociology of Education, 22*(4), 445–461.

Mykhalovskiy, E., & Weir, L. (2004). The problem of evidence-based medicine: Directions for social science. *Social Science and Medicine, 59*(5), 1059–1069.

Naidoo, R., & Jamieson, I. (2005). Empowering participants or corroding learning? Towards a research agenda on the impact of student consumerism in higher education. *Journal of Educational Policy, 20*(3), 267–281.

Nelson, R., & Ball, M. J. (2003). Models of phonology in the education of speech-language pathologists. *Clinical Linguistics & Phonetics, 17*(4–5), 403–409.

Oakley, A. (2006). Resistances to "new" technologies of evaluation: Education research in the UK as a case study. *Evidence & Policy, 2*(1), 63–87.

Packman, A., Rousseau, I., Onslow, M., Dredge, R., Harrison, E., & Wilson, L. (2003). Part IV: The Lidcombe Program around the world. In M. Onslow, A. Packman, & E. Harrison (Eds.), *The Lidcombe Program of early stuttering intervention: A clinician's guide* (pp. 139–146). Austin, TX: Pro-Ed.

Pillay, M., Kathard, H., & Samuel, M. A. (1997). The curriculum of practice: A conceptual framework for speech-language therapy and audiology practice with a Black African first language clientele. *South African Journal of Communication Disorders, 44,* 109–117.

Prince, K. J. A., Boshuizen, H. P. A., Van der Vleuten, C. P. M., & Scherpbier, A. J. J. A. (2005). Students' opinions about their preparation for clinical practice. *Medical Education, 39,* 704–712.

Reilly, S., Douglas, J., & Oates, J. (Eds.). (2004). *Evidence based practice in speech pathology.* London: Whurr.

Reilly, S., Oates, J., & Douglas, J. (2004). Evidence-based practice in speech pathology—future directions. In S. Reilly, J. Douglas, & J. Oates (Eds.), *Evidence based practice in speech pathology* (pp. 330–352). London: Whurr.

Robley, W., Whittle, S., & Murdoch-Eaton, D. (2005). Mapping generic skills curricula: Outcomes and discussion. *Journal of Further and Higher Education, 29*(4), 321–330.

Rose, M., & Baldac, S. (2004). Translating evidence into practice. In S. Reilly, J. Douglas, & J. Oates (Eds.), *Evidence based practice in speech pathology* (pp. 317–329). London: Whurr.

Rose, M. L. (2005). The cycle of crisis in clinical education: Why national-level strategies must be prioritized. *Advances in Speech-Language Pathology, 7*(3), 158–161.

Sackett, D. L., Straus, S. E., Richardson, W. S., Rosenberg, W., & Haynes, R. B. (2000). *Evidence-based medicine: How to practice and teach EBM.* Edinburgh: Churchill Livingstone.

Siegel, G. M., & Ingham, R. J. (1987). Theory and science in communication disorders. *Journal of Speech & Hearing Disorders, 52,* 99–104.

Stewart, S. R., & Gonzalez, L. S. (2002). Serving a diverse population: The role of speech-language pathology professional preparation programs. *Journal of Allied Health, 31*(4), 204–216.

Stiwne, D., & Dahlgren, M. A. (2004). Challenging evidence in evidence-based practice. In J. Higgs, B. Richardson, & M. A. Dahlgren (Eds.), *Developing practice knowledge for health professionals* (pp. 147–164). Edinburgh: Butterworth Heinemann.

Stockman, I. J., Boult, J., & Robinson, G. (2004, July). Multicultural issues in academic and clinical education: A cultural mosaic. *ASHA Leader,* 6–7, 20–22.

Talbot, M. (2004). Monkey see, monkey do: A critique of the competency model in graduate medical education. *Medical Education, 38,* 587–592.

Tanenbaum, S. (2003). Evidence-based practice in mental health: Practical weaknesses meet political strengths. *Journal of Evaluation in Clinical Practice, 9*(2), 287–301.

Tanner, D., & Tanner, L. (2007). Changing conceptions of curriculum. In *Curriculum development: Theory into practice* (pp. 98–123). Upper Saddle River, NJ: Pearson Merrill/Pearson Hall.

Tastle, W. J., White, B. A., & Shackleton, P. (2005). E-learning in higher education: The challenge, effort, and return on investment. *International Journal on ELearning, 4*(2), 241–251.

Yaruss, J. S., & Quesal, R. W. (2002). Academic and clinical education in fluency disorders: An update. *Journal of Fluency Disorders, 27,* 43–63.

Young, M. F. D. (1971). An approach to the study of curricula as a socially organized knowledge. In M. F. D. Young (Ed.), *Knowledge and social control: New directions for the sociology of education* (pp. 19–46). London: Collier-Macmillan.

9

Future Directions from a Critical Discourse Perspective

Discourse Perpetuates and Creates Culture

This chapter examines the perspective of critical discourse analysis and argues that the contribution of this perspective to expert speech-language pathology practice is its capacity to promote alternative directions for research and change in the profession. In particular, two of the issues very familiar to speech-language pathologists are examined: the socio-cultural homogeneity of the profession and the general lack of public awareness regarding communication disorders and of the role of the profession.

Critique of the Critical Discourse Perspective

Some of the criticisms that can be made with regard to the critical discourse perspective relate to the wider post-modern theoretical paradigm (e.g., critique with regard to its sociological constructs, with regard to both culture and power). Other issues are of direct concern to the perspective itself (e.g., critique with regard to its methodologies and scope of application).

Relationship of Discourse with Culture: Inadequate Theory

The critical discourse perspective has been critiqued with regard to the inadequate theoretical base in relation to sociological theory for constructs of culture and society. So although the critical discourse perspective in general and the specific approaches for critical discourse analysis involving, for example, systemic functional linguistics, rely heavily on notions of social context, neither the analytical method nor the related approaches are articulated or integrated within wider sociological theories of power (for example, both refer to gender or class, but without reference to how these operate) (J. B. Thompson, 1984). Also, Widdowson has criticized critical discourse analysis in terms of its preoccupation with relatively small stretches of text on which rather large claims rest in relation to social context: "The process whereby these forms interrelate co-textually with each other and contextually with the circumstances of their use is left largely unexplored. Text is treated as a kind of static semantic patchwork, existing as an object for analysis in its own right" (Widdowson, 2000, p. 22). Bartlett (2004), however, argues that this insufficiency reflects the early stages of development of the approaches (both critical discourse analysis and systemic functional linguistics), rather than being intrinsic to them. In other words, further theoretical development is needed with regard to how the approaches characterize the interrelationship of discourse and culture. Nevertheless, an important point to be explored is whether critical discourse perspectives need (or aim) to provide a unified and complete theoretical account, or whether the contribution is chiefly as a vantage point from which the social nature of discourse can be viewed, with an accompanying methodology for mapping this terrain.

Relationship of Discourse with Cognition: Inadequate Theory

Chilton (2005) argues that critical discourse analysis has been selectively interdisciplinary in its close ties with sociology and philosophy, so that as an important disciplinary tool it has failed to take into account more recent developments in cognitive psychology. In particular, Chilton suggests that cognitive psychology, in its developments of such constructs as "theory of mind" and social cognition for group behavior, has offered ways by which people's sociocultural experience becomes mapped within mental representations. He suggests that critical discourse analysis fails to acknowledge or consider the ways in which mental representations encode sociocultural phenomena. Speech-language pathologists, on the other hand, work from a theoretical base that is widely interdisciplinary and will readily recognize the social-individual linkages to which Chilton draws attention; for example, refer to the discussion in Chapter 1 regarding the relevance of Van Dijk's work to understandings of mental schema as they relate to sociocultural experience (Van Dijk, 2006; Van Dijk & Kintsch, 1983). It can be suggested, then, that speech-language pathologists are well placed to further the development of the theoretical base for critical discourse perspectives and the development of social mental representations and the critical self.

Sociocultural Discourse Learning: Insufficiently Explored

Although the critical discourse perspective has been influential in the field of education, such perspectives have been criticized for paying insufficient attention to learning (and this criticism relates to the previous point with regard to cognition and its development). Accordingly, many educationalists and researchers have drawn on the work of sociocultural learning theorists such as Vygotsky in order to supply this lack (Rowe, 2004)—and indeed, this is the approach taken in this book (see Chapter 7). On the other hand, Fairclough (2004) argues that a critical discourse framework does enable an understanding of social learning, and his view is premised on the view of individual learning as reflecting sociocultural understandings through transmission by means of discourse. Certainly, further research is needed in order to explore sociocultural discourse learning, but whether critical discourse analysis can or should offer a single perspective with regard to learning is questionable. As discussed earlier in relation to sociological theory, the wealth of theoretical understandings available from other perspectives that are compatible with a critical discourse framework must prompt the suggestion that here too, critical discourse analysis offers a perspective and methodology to assist in the exploration of this territory.

Relationship of Discourse with Action: Insufficiently Recognized

From a critical discourse perspective, it sometimes can appear that all interaction is composed of discourse, to the exclusion of the world of activity and action. Some approaches seek to develop an understanding of the integration of discourse and action—for example, "mediated discourse analysis" (Norris & Jones, 2005). Such approaches arguably go beyond the

scope currently offered by systemic functional linguistics in capturing the world of action. In speech-language pathology professional practice, interaction is both discourse *and* action: The discourse of assessment sets up the constraints for understanding of the discourse of people with communication disorders, and the therapeutic medium to facilitate discourse understanding and production is itself discourse. This interrelationship between discourse and action is thus of vital concern to speech-language pathology practice, and further development of critical discourse analysis is needed to assist this exploration.

Analysis of Discourse: Contradictory Paradigms?

Critical discourse perspectives embody an apparent paradox: Such perspectives are informed from postmodern and interpretive paradigms, yet the associated primary research methodologies can be argued to be essentially positivist or scientific in nature. These methodologies have been seen to be valuable to critical discourse analysis in its own disciplinary power struggle to be seen as legitimate, so, for example, the systematic and textually grounded approach offered by systemic functional linguistics has offered a "scientific" way to approach the critical task. Through adoption of such top-down methodologies, however, as noted by Widdowson (2000), the focus on textual analysis plus the privileging of researcher interpretations over that of participants prevents access to the value of interactants' perceptions and meanings. Although he concurs with the importance of the critical purpose of critical discourse analysis, Widdowson argues for the greater validity of more ethnographic approaches, particularly in the application of linguistics in the application to everyday problem-solving. His concerns are rebutted by de Beaugrande (2001), particularly with regard to some fundamental misinterpretations of methodologies used, but the central tension remains about who is doing the interpreting. As discussed in Chapter 1, when the positivist approach was criticized for the researcher domination of interpretation, so too must critical discourse analysis be open to the same criticism when it is done without reference to multiple perspectives and points of interpretation (but see the caveats on triangulation in Chapter 2). Hammersley concurs with this critique, which he sees as applicable not only to discourse analysis approaches (such as systemic functional linguistics) but also to the ethnomethodological approach of conversation analysis (Hammersley, 2003). For example, conversation analysis purports to use participants' perspectives, but the participants' accounts *are* data in this approach and therefore subject to researcher analysis, and discourse analysis claims that researchers are participants within the same societal discourse as that of interactants (and hence offer participant accounts). It is not possible, however, to verify such interpretations (because, through the internal logic of the approach, the interactants' interpretations are seen as intrinsically subject to social construction).

This apparent paradox can be resolved if it is recognized that critical or postmodern approaches are not necessarily "anti-science"—as Skrtic (1995)

observes, the issues revolve around the recognition of the sociopolitical processes involved in the conduct of science. As described by Kuhn (1970) in his work on paradigm shifts in science, much of science progresses in much the way in which the positivist paradigm suggests, that is, cumulatively and objectively, but major breakthroughs entailing paradigm shifts occur through social processes. Thus, scientific and critical perspectives need not be set up as a binary opposition; instead, the objective conduct of everyday science can itself be seen as occurring within a particular cultural framework. So, just as scientific practices are useful in practice and research, they are useful in the conduct of critical discourse analysis, but it also is important to recognize the social processes and cultural frameworks that are driving and shaping the work, respectively. One of the functions of critical approaches within linguistics is to generate theory and questions regarding the nature of suitable problems for the application of linguistic theory to real-world problem-solving and, in doing so, to generate the ethical debate in relation to the wider sociocultural and sociopolitical contexts of applied linguistics (Carlson, 2004; Kress, 1990).

Relationship of Discourse and Power: Explanation or Focus?

Within critical perspectives, the notion of power and its relationship with discourse is variously construed. As Gaventa and Cornwall (2001) observe, for some theorists, *power* is essentially negatively construed (such as in much of the work of Fairclough)—for example, in the issue of who is considered the expert to be consulted in sociopolitical decision-making, or as necessarily involving conflict (between the powerful and the powerless), or as controlled through processes of socialization (such as education, media). From this view, power is the explanation for inequitable distribution of information, goods, and services. For those working from a foucauldian approach, however, power is relational—the power to act. Thus, for example, Foucault saw power as producing knowledge within society and, at the same time, saw knowledge as being productive of power: "L'exercice du pouvoir crée perpétuellement du savoir et inversement, le savoir entraîne des effects de pouvoir" (Foucault, 2001, p. 1620). From this perspective, power can be seen as operating in all aspects of social relations, working through the discourses, institutions, and practices of the society. Power is itself the object of study: "I've never claimed that power was going to explain everything . . . For me, power is what needs to be explained" (Foucault, 2000, p. 284). This latter approach argues that critical awareness of the network of social power relations allows for understanding of constraints as well as providing means for social change.

Discourse Analysis and Problem-Solving: Reflection or Action?

As previously discussed in this book, one of the common criticisms of critical postmodern perspectives is that if all perspectives are seen as of equal value, then how can judgments be made regarding directions to follow? The danger of the critical perspective is that reflection can lead to despair or impotence, rather than leading to hope for improvement and effective action.

For those working within the critical perspective, the approach does not set out to solve problems, because to do so would be to assume that, first, there is a "right" way to proceed and, second, the researcher is the one who knows the right way. Instead, the critical perspective seeks to *problematize*, in the sense of bringing the issues involved out into the open (Pennycook, 2001, pp. 41–43). From such problematizing discussions, all sorts of consequences may result, including insight or awareness, directions for further investigation, and direct action. This process is framed deliberately to avoid "power-play" while aiming for change. Thus, the researcher is seen as having the social responsibility for raising issues but not as the professional agent who should say whether change should occur and, if so, how or what should change.

For many, the perspective offered by Habermas provides a midway path through the issues raised by critical theory. As Kemmis (2001) describes it, the Habermas perspective has been applied productively to educational research, perhaps because it recognizes different ways in which critical research can proceed while still being action-oriented research. Thus, for example, problem-solving research can be mainly technical in terms of its goals to improve patient outcomes, whereas research aiming to inform professional practice at the same time as improving patient outcomes can be largely practical ("communicative," "pragmatic") in its goals, but some action research can be "emancipatory," in which more critical awareness and questioning of the bases of the goals themselves can occur. Ethical issues for research with this sort of agenda are well recognized—as Johnston (2000) observes, can research really be participatory when researchers are providing emancipation? Although researchers may hold emancipatory goals, Kemmis notes that " . . . others cannot do the enlightening for participants; in the end, they are or are not enlightened in their own terms" (p. 91). In other words, the critical approach offers a lever, a tool, a method, but the actual revelations and change constitute a product of the approach.

As research that seeks to problematize, critical discourse analysis always comes with the possibility that findings and outcomes may be contrary to those anticipated and may be discomforting to researchers, participants, funding agencies, and consumers of the research. As discussed in Chapter 1, critical discourse analysis is risky business, but its potential for offering alternative perspectives and directions for change is considerable, and just some of these possibilities with regard to expert speech-language pathology practice are discussed in the next section.

Research Agenda

In this section, the main themes from each chapter in this book are revisited to identify some of the main directions for further research from a critical discourse perspective into expert speech-language pathology practice. Any of numerous methodologies may be em-

ployed in such research, but certainly participatory action research provides a methodological framework that is well suited to be integrated with critical discourse analysis for such research (Reason & Bradbury, 2001).

The Discourse of Scope of Practice

From the outset of this book, the notion of discourse as a reflection of culture has been discussed in relation to the scope of practice in speech-language pathology. Through the analysis of the discourse of the profession in relation to scope of practice in Chapter 1, speech-language pathology was clearly identified as a profession that has invested heavily in the scientific positivist paradigm. Expert speech-language pathology practice can be seen to be about applying interpretive judgments with regard to appropriateness of communication, while at the same time using the apparent objectivity of science as a warrant for these judgments. From a critical discourse perspective, more research is needed to examine the role of speech-language pathologists as both gatekeepers and gateways to services for people with communication and swallowing disorders. In what ways do speech-language pathologists act as agents of institutions (such as education and health), or alternatively, to empower persons or groups of persons within society? How are wider social inequalities (such as class, gender, and those associated with geographical isolation) reflected in speech-language pathology practice? More fundamentally, what are the issues faced by expert speech-language pathologists when the demands of institutions and clients are conflicting, and what processes are involved in attempts to resolve these conflicts?

The Discourse of Assessment

In making judgments regarding appropriateness of communication, expert speech-language pathologists draw on assessment methodologies that are both quantitative and qualitative in nature; in both approaches, an understanding of the context of communication is essential. In formal, standardized assessments, significant aspects of context need to be identified and systematically controlled, whereas informal assessments intrinsically entail an exploration of discourse within natural contexts. In Chapter 2, the multilayered relationship between discourse and the contexts in which it is produced was explored, in order to consider from a critical perspective the issues of validity that arise during assessment. Expert speech-language pathologists need to make practical decisions on a daily basis, so a critical discourse perspective would assist in understanding more about how they do (or do not) integrate such competing approaches to assessment. Moreover, expert speech-language pathologists are likely to design assessments in light of what they already perceive as the end-goal for client management (that is, assessments are purpose-driven), so a greater understanding is needed with regard to what influences their determination of goals for intervention. In particular, the sociopolitical context of assessment requires consid-

eration at all times by practitioners, in order to recognize where, for example, political and economic agenda are being served by assessment practices.

The Discourse of Decision-Making

Little is known about how expert speech-language pathologists make their assessment decisions, and Chapter 3 looked at three examples that typically are identified as challenging in professional practice: medicolegal, higher-level language, and bilingual assessment. As noted, each of these processes of assessment requires informal assessment practices, reflecting the dynamic nature of discourse (which is affected by changes in aspects of context, including temporal aspects). Despite the apparent paradox (similar to that discussed earlier in this chapter), the positivist decision-making process may provide an explicit method to assist the interpretive judgments about cultural context required in such complex assessments. Further research is required to deconstruct the everyday decision-making of expert speech-language pathologists in conducting complex assessments, in order to illuminate both the reasoning and the cultural influences involved.

The Discourse of Empowerment and Advocacy

The view of speech-language pathology services differs for the client and for the clinician, and Chapter 4 explored the differences between the narratives for each. The notions of collaboration and partnership were considered critically, and the power relations, although asymmetrical, were presented as potentially productive for people with communication disorders. The critical issues in relation to advocacy centered on the extent to which professionals could or should advocate on behalf of clients; instead, adoption of approaches through which client self-advocacy could be promoted was suggested as a productive direction. More research that highlights the voices of people with communication disorders about their lives and their experiences with the profession would greatly illuminate issues with regard to both the scope and the nature of practice. Further research is needed in relation to the issues of scope of practice with regard to advocacy, and specifically with regard to the processes by which empowerment can be facilitated.

The Discourse of Collaboration

Working collaboratively with professionals from other disciplines was discussed in Chapter 5, with reference not only to the discourse that occurs in face-to-face interaction but also to the intersections and misconnections between disciplinary and institutional discourses. Further research is needed at the level of face-to-face interaction between professionals from different professions, because this level has immediate effects on the management of people with communication disorders, particularly with reference to their access to services. Further research also is needed with regard to the similarities and differences between professional discourses, and how these differences

play out in institutional practices (and also how these resultant practices affect services to people with communication disorders).

The Discourse of Therapy

The genres of speech-language pathology practice were discussed in Chapter 6, mainly with reference to the "session." The recognition of the systematic, organized, and predictable nature of such types of discourse leads to the identification of the ways in which such discourse can be both exploited (for example, by experts for therapeutic ends) and learned (for example, by novices entering the profession). Further research is needed in order to develop more understanding of the social construction of identity as "client" and "clinician," and how this construction may be related to particular aspects or elements of the therapeutic process, rather than the session itself.

Learning the Discourse

Chapter 7 explored the interactional processes through which the discourse associated with expert speech-language pathology practice is learned. That chapter identified discourse bridges to expertise and examined the role of critical awareness as fundamental to the process of learning through the use of these bridges. Further research is needed into these processes of learning, not just into expert-learner interactions but also more fundamentally into how learners construct their understandings as a result of their hands-on experience.

Teaching the Discourse

The discourse of speech-language pathology practice is enshrined institutionally through curriculum, and Chapter 8 examined the role of curriculum development and delivery as a tool for cultural reproduction of the profession. As an answer to the potential for "cloning" through the cultural reproduction of education, the role of critical perspectives in education may be to provide for cultural production (creation) of lifelong learning skills that enable learners to think beyond the perspectives of their educators. Evidence-based practice and research as a discourse within the profession were critiqued; and although some limitations were identified, this approach also was argued to be important to add to the understanding of how curriculum can be delivered effectively, and such benchmarking research is in its infancy. The theory-practice issues that are fundamental to applied disciplines such as speech-language pathology were seen as potentially benefiting from further research into how the discourse needed within employing institutions can be taught within educational discourse. Furthermore, research into the ways in which the perspectives of people with communication disorders can shape curriculum and learning outcomes is needed.

The Discourse of Cultural and Linguistic Diversity

Throughout this book, the issues associated with cultural and linguistic diversity have been recognized as per-

tinent to every aspect of professional practice. In Chapter 3, the issues associated with bilingual assessment were discussed; in Chapter 5, the issues that arise in interpreter-mediated sessions were considered. In both of these chapters, cultural and linguistic diversity was presented as an issue that would benefit greatly from being "problematized," rather than as a difficulty to be overcome. Although much of the research and professional literature in this area takes the form of exhortations for equity and prescriptions for what needs to be done, little has changed. Instead, research is needed from a critical discourse perspective to examine the issues for all involved (for example, what do people from cultural and linguistically diverse backgrounds expect or want from speech-language pathologists?). In Chapters 7 and 8, speech-language pathology students from cultural and linguistically diverse backgrounds were identified as a resource for clients, clinicians, and other students. Although such students too often are seen as a problem for educators, further research from a critical discourse perspective would enable a wider view of the issues involved and would promote the recognition that even the labeling of such difference involves a process of "other-ing," rather than a recognition of the universality of intercultural communication issues.

Analyzing the Discourse

Although at times in this book particular textual analyses and examples have been presented in order to illustrate points made, this book is but an overview of some of the territory yet to be explored. As previously mentioned, participatory action research appears well suited to the type of research suggested as needing further exploration (Reason & Bradbury, 2001), and although some researchers working from critical discourse perspectives would argue for a purist approach to methodology, a wide range of approaches currently are seen in the published research in this area. Many researchers adopt a mixed-methodology approach, which has the advantage of requiring explicit articulation of purposes with methods (Creswell, 2003), rather than adoption through habitual practice, familiarity, or paradigmatic constraints. Within such a mixed-methodology approach, researchers may adopt quantitative hypothesis-driven scientific approaches as a useful methodology, particularly for matters in which the main constructs are well identified. Qualitative interpretive approaches using ethnographic or narrative methodologies are well suited to exploring new territory, particularly in research seeking the perspectives of others. Consistent with such an ethnographic approach, conversation analysis methodology is useful for exploring interactions in terms of broad interactional features (such as turn-taking, hesitation phenomena, and laughter) and is free of any particular a priori theoretical assumptions about how such observations should necessarily be interpreted (Prevignano & Thibault, 2003). Although a range of approaches are possible with discourse analysis (Coulthard, 1992), the approach most closely associated with critical research is that of systemic functional linguistics, in keeping with its focus on the relationship of language and particular aspects of context

(Young & Harrison, 2004). Systemic functional linguistic analyses allow for a close description of lexicogrammar (which is unavailable through conversation analysis), and the approach is suited to the analysis of both interactional data and monologic narrative data, in both spoken and written forms (Butt, Fahey, Feez, Spinks, & Yallop, 2000; Eggins, 1994; Eggins & Slade, 2004/1997; Halliday & Matthiessen, 2004; Martin, Matthiessen, & Painter, 1997; Martin & Rose, 2003; Matthiessen & Halliday, 1997; G. Thompson, 1996). These theoretical and methodological aspects of systemic functional linguistic analyses provide considerable resources for the conduct of critical discourse analysis.

Action Agenda

Although many directions for further research are recognized, a critical discourse perspective also can illuminate multiple directions for action. The most apparent directions for action that emerge from this book relate to the cultural instantiation of the profession, which is closely related to the awareness of speech-language pathology in society, and who enters the profession (which of course is related to the wider cultural awareness issues).

Chapter 1 made clear that the scope of practice documents of the profession are designed for use in situations in which the nature of the profession's populations and types of work needs to be communicated to those outside the profession. In these documents, the populations and types of work that are well recognized by the general public receive relatively less specific attention than those that are less well recognized —for example, specific caveats are made with regard to evaluation of esophageal function. In this book, however, it has been argued that identity is socially constructed—that is, it is through the relationship with others that identity comes into being. Cultural identity, therefore, is defined not by how the profession defines practice but by how others view communication and swallowing disorders and the role of speech-language pathologists. In the following discussion of these issues, public awareness of communication disorders is considered first, followed by public awareness of the role of the profession.

Public Awareness of Communication Disorder

In considering the social construct of communication disorder, it is helpful to separate for the moment the wider issues regarding how communication disorders are viewed and understood in society from the issues associated with public awareness of particular labels or terminology used to describe these phenomena.

Communication disorders have existed throughout human history but, as noted by O'Neill (1980), have been viewed very differently depending on the sociocultural influences associated with particular epochs. For example, according to this researcher, competence in communication was fundamental to the concept of humanness in Western thought in the pre-Renaissance period, so loss of speech and language was seen as diminishing this quality, with resulting differential treatment. Such

social constructs are so embedded within the culture that it can be difficult to identify them and see how they operate in current society. The work of Preston (1996) is relevant here: He notes that folk perceptions of language differ from linguists' perceptions, as seen on a continuum of linguistic awareness and the extent to which it can be consciously available or retrievable. Applying these ideas to the awareness of communication disorders would suggest that, for example, stuttering is very "available" in the sense that people talk about it and identify it without prompting, and that although lay descriptions of stuttering are not specific descriptions, most people can manage reasonable performance of imitated stuttering. This level of availability is in contrast with that for aphasic verbal expression, which can be suggested to be very "unavailable" for most people (unless perhaps they have personal familiarity). Aphasic verbal expression is unlikely to come up in general conversation, and lay descriptions tend to be very general descriptions and differ from those of speech-language pathologists, and apart from word-finding difficulty, many aspects of aphasic verbal expression (agrammatism, extended jargon) are difficult to imitate. Preston suggests that folk perspectives tend to describe language difference prescriptively in terms of deviation from one perceived correct standard, in contrast to the way linguists seek to identify patterns and rule-governed systems over many deviations. With regard to communication disorder, then, the folk perception identifies and stigmatizes difference, because the default folk assumption is that all speakers have access to the one system. As Preston notes, however, people do not detect or note every difference for a speaker; rather, the differences they identify tend to be cultural stereotypes and caricatures. Preston suggests that the cultural and communications media contribute greatly to the production of such stereotypes but also that the media constitute an extension of the more pervasive social processes involved in identification of social groupings and differences in relation to social power in the culture, such as occurs with dialectal identity, for example. Certainly with regard to communication disorders, the media reflect the wider societal caricatures associated with, for instance, the exploitation of stuttering and lateral "s" for humorous purposes (e.g., in the speech of Porky Pig and Daffy Duck, respectively) or the association of dysphonia with "sexy" voice or of hyponasality with intellectual limitations. This state of awareness of communication disorder is the very stuff that is handicapping on a day-to-day basis for people with communication disorders and is the most powerfully culturally embedded. It may be that personal familiarity with people with communication disorders is the main way in which members of the public break away from such stereotypes. For example, Killarney and Lass (1981) conducted a telephone survey of 200 people in a rural location; roughly half of the survey participants knew people with either speech-language or hearing problems. The role of the media, then, can be seen as supplying such exposure to people without personal familiarity with someone with a communication disorder.

Labeling of communication disorders within the community reflects the more embedded social construction of the differences from the folk perception of standard or competent communication. With increasing frequency, publications in the discipline are calling for improved consistency in speech-language pathologists' use of terminology within the community of practice, as an important step to communicate more effectively with the general public about various patterns of difference (Eadie, 2005). As Duchan notes, the speech-language pathology profession historically has adopted Latin forms for diagnostic labeling, in line with the profession's strong medical affiliation (see the discussion in Chapter 8 regarding the way new disciplines attach to high-status established disciplines in their establishment period)—for example, "dyslalia," "dysphagia" (J. F. Duchan, 2004). Most public awareness surveys in the profession have focused on the awareness of such labels and their meaning (rather than on the actual nature of communication disorder and how it is perceived). For example, a recent survey researched the recognition of the term *aphasia* across 929 people in three countries: the United States, the United Kingdom, and Australia (Code et al., 2001; Simmons-Mackie, Code, Armstrong, Stiegler, & Elman, 2002). Although 10% to 18% of persons in the sample had heard the term, fewer knew what it involved (1.5% to 7.6%). Roughly one third reported that their knowledge about aphasia came from the media, and approximately one third reported that the term came up at work. Although females were more likely than men to recognize the term, this appeared to be related to contact with the condition through the nature of their work. On the basis of such research, increasing attention has been given to raising general awareness of the term *aphasia* as a means of increasing public support for persons with this communication disorder.

But will awareness solve the problems faced by people with communication disorders? Stuttering is a good example of a communication disorder that has widespread social recognition (as opposed to, say, aphasia); nevertheless, the social perception of persons with this impairment is as a highly negative stereotype, with undesirable attributes such being excessively shy or anxious (Daniels & Gabel, 2004). As Goffman points out, a "spread" of disability occurs such that problems observed in one aspect of function are assumed to affect other aspects of function (Goffman, 1968). Such stigmatizing cultural stereotyping is very powerful, resulting, in the case of stuttering, for example, in discrimination and restricted opportunities in employment and education as well as in social interactions (Daniels & Gabel, 2004). The awareness of such cultural stereotypes affects the lives of people with communication disorders both directly and indirectly, so that they may come to anticipate such stigmatizing—and this anticipation itself can lead to self-imposed restrictions (Klein & Hood, 2004). Speech-language pathology as a profession has tended to tackle such issues as cultural stereotyping through directing intervention toward empowerment of persons with communication disorders. For example, Daniels and Gabel (2004) suggest a therapy approach

modeled on Hagstrom and Wertsch's ideas about mediated action in which therapy aims to give affected persons the cultural tools to handle the problem in their interactions with other people (Hagstrom & Wertsch, 2004). Although such suggestions are important ways forward, they locate the direction of intervention at the affected person's interaction with members of society, when the clearer need is for ways to shift wider community perceptions. Endeavors to shift societal constructs of communication disorder could make use of the processes applied in other areas of disability to achieve increased public awareness, such as the work being done with regard to mental health and attempts to destigmatize mental illness.

Raising public awareness requires a degree of shared community among people with similar communication problems, and this sense of shared community is not always present, and may in fact not always be desirable for individuals. In considering such issues as relating to awareness of disability from a cultural perspective, Deal (2003) notes that cultural stereotypes are both sociohistorical and developmental. For example, young children tend to be more accepting of difference, but as they start to need to identify with a particular group, then culturally acquired notions begin to appear.

People with acquired disability face a cultural identity shift, because their attitudes toward their disabled self may reflect attitudes to that disability before injury. Regardless of societal identification, particular groups may not identify as a disabled group (for example, "deaf," as opposed to "hearing-impaired"), and some affected persons may reject disabled group membership either because of the perceived nature of the problem (Parr, Byng, Gilpin, & Ireland, 1997) or as a result of cultural conceptions of the problem (Salas-Provance, Erickson, & Reed, 2002). The movement in speech-language pathology toward advocating for greater public awareness of particular types of communication disorder reflects recent moves in the social disability movement toward greater differentiation among subgroups of disability (Deal, pp. 902-903). The benefits are seen in terms of increasing the level of community support (for example, funding for services and research), but the risks need to be recognized regarding increasing competition for scarce resources, rather than expanding the resource base. Elman and colleagues, for example, talk about the political and economic consequences of public awareness in relation to aphasia, noting that funding for services and for research does not relate to incidence disorder in the population but rather reflects the extent of political visibility in the community (Elman, Ogar, & Elman, 2000). Increased "brand recognition" associated with specific labeling of communication disorders helps with political and governmental recognition, as can be seen in the case of the government-mandated provision of services in U.S. schools (Pickering et al., 1998).

This recognition of the potential power of socially recognized labels for communication disorders works against much of what people with communication disorders and speech-pathologists are trying to achieve—that is, acceptance of difference as normal, not abnormal. The link to the medical label renders the disorder important in a world that values science and yet makes the problem due to something other than the the the affected person's fault and thus a situation requiring individual empathy and community support. By using medical labels and promoting their widespread adoption through the community, are speech-language pathologists helping or hindering? Is it possible to increase public awareness without further stigmatizing people with communication disorders? One way forward from a critical discourse perspective is to explore public understandings of communication disorders, in a fashion similar to that advocated by Lupton (1992) for the field of public health more generally—that is, through the exploration of public discourse. Part of such a research direction would involve the exploration of how people talk about communication disorder in conversational interaction but, in view of the role of the media in shaping cultural familiarity, also would involve a deeper look at media messages to understand public understandings. Elman and colleagues' (2000) research represents a first step in this direction. These investigators looked at 50 of the 352 newspaper stories mentioning aphasia that had appeared in the previous 5 years in 50 leading U.S. newspapers. In 20 of the 50 stories, no explanation of the term was given; in 17, a short definition was provided; and in only 13 was significant content provided in relation to the disorder and its effects on people's lives. Left unexplored was the nature of the mentions in the far more numerous stories on the other conditions considered in the study (Parkinson's disease, stuttering, multiple sclerosis, autism, and muscular dystrophy). Such a critical discourse perspective could inform directions for change by identifying what sorts of stories receive the widest distribution and the deepest coverage.

Public Awareness of the Speech-Language Pathology Profession

The history of the speech-language pathology profession is brief, particularly when it is considered that the first professionals working with people with communication disorders in Western culture (both Europe and the United States), during the late nineteenth century, came from a range of other professional backgrounds—for example, both education and medical backgrounds (J. Duchan, 2002; J. F. Duchan, 2004). The speech-language pathology profession formed a professional association in the United States in the mid-1920s, and Eldridge (1968) suggests that the discipline came to be recognized as an independent profession in the 1930s, with considerable expansion occurring subsequently as a result of an increasing role of rehabilitation during and after World War II.

In the public awareness survey by Killarney and Lass (1981) mentioned previously, of 200 respondents, 54% recognized *speech pathologist* or *speech therapist* as the professional working with speech or language problems, and none were able to identify the professional association. Using a similar telephone survey, Parsons and colleagues interviewed 400 Australians (Parsons, Bowman, & Iacono, 1983). Although 41% of respondents did not identify the profession when asked "What would/

do you call the professional who provides training for people who have speech, language, or communication problems?" 83% reported that they had heard any of the terms *speech therapist, speech pathologist,* and *speech clinician*. In other words, "brand recognition" for the profession appears to be higher than the community understanding of the nature of the work associated with the speech-language pathology profession. Certainly, in a market survey in Australia, one third of 300 Australians interviewed were reported as not recognizing what speech pathology involved (*Survey report on general public perceptions on speech pathology and its meaning,* 1995). Similarly, in the United Kingdom, one third of 651 school students (around 16 to 17 years of age) reported that they knew nothing about speech and language therapy (Greenwood, Wright, & Bithell, 2006), and some of the subset of 11 interviewees commented that the profession was not portrayed in the media, for example, on medical dramas on television. As with public awareness of communication disorders, as discussed previously, it can be suggested that the issues related to labeling of the profession are important for their sociopolitical purposes but can distract from the more fundamental issues regarding the ability of members of the community to know when they need a speech-language pathologist, and where and how to obtain speech-language pathology services (and, of course, how to become one; see later section in this chapter).

Even within related professions, awareness of the role of speech-language pathologists has been found to be less than ideal. Lesser and Hassip (1986), in a study of awareness of speech-language pathology in physicians, nurses, and teachers (both as students and as qualified professionals), found that all groups (33 in each group) identified speech-language pathologists as working with persons with stuttering and cleft palate, but changes in scope of practice incorporating work with dementia, literacy, and pediatric feeding were not reflected in their awareness. A surprising finding was that the related professionals were less likely than speech-language pathology students and professionals to associate voice disorders, laryngectomy, and cerebral palsy with speech-language pathology practice but were more likely to associate deafness with the profession. Continuing problems with the strong association of the term *elocution* and the profession was reported, but Lesser and Hassip note that this term may reflect lay nomenclature for working with articulation (p. 244).

A study by Sullivan and Cleave (2003) used an alternative methodology that enabled them to move away from the labeling dilemma when looking at what 268 students from medicine, nursing, occupational therapy, and physiotherapy knew about the roles of speech-language pathologists. Their method involved presenting the students with 18 short case studies of disorders of which 13 typically would involve a speech-language pathologist (global developmental delay, cleft palate, apraxia, cerebral palsy, laryngeal cancer, Down syndrome, language delay, voice, Alzheimer's disease, swallowing, autism, right hemisphere stroke, and traumatic brain injury). The students then were asked to select three professionals from a list who might be involved in the case apart from the

family doctor. In a comparison of first- and final-year students, all students except those from medicine showed significantly more knowledge by the end of their programs, with the biggest change associated with recognition of swallowing. The students showed the highest awareness of speech-language pathologists' work with developmental delay and cleft palate, and the lowest awareness of their work with traumatic brain injury (only 4%). Further research could employ a similar methodology to explore public awareness of the profession. In view of the suggested relationship between awareness and access to services (O'Callaghan, McAllister, & Wilson, 2005), it also would be important to consider public awareness research and direction of action strategies toward those groups within society that traditionally appear to receive inequitable service provision (such as rural or remote, indigenous, and other culturally and linguistically diverse populations).

Who Decides to be a Speech-Language Pathologist—and Why?

Throughout this book, the homogeneity of the speech-language pathology profession has been a recurring issue, affecting the extent of understanding of issues for client groups and scope of practice itself. Homogeneity can be seen to confer advantage to the profession in many ways, such as in contributing to the cohesion within the community of practice, but does raise the question of whether alternative viewpoints and practices exist or could be developed to better fit provision of services for diverse populations. One of the ways that has been suggested to diversify practice within the profession has been to attend to recruitment strategies through which students enter speech-language pathology professional education programs.

The social demographic profile of the speech-language pathology profession is overwhelmingly middle class, altruism-driven, female, and white (Stewart, Pool, & Winn, 2002). For example, with regard to social class, in a study of 43 speech-language pathology students compared with students in other allied health programs, Nordholm and Westbrook (1978) found that all allied health students came from predominantly upper middle and middle class backgrounds (based on the father's occupation). With regard to issues related to altruism, Adamson and colleagues looked at personality attributes in speech in students studying speech-language pathology and medical radiation science (Adamson, Covic, Kench, & Lincoln, 2003). These investigators found no significant difference between these two groups, with both falling into the personality types described as guardians and idealists ("concerned citizens") with the ability to identify with others. Even the roughly one third of students who were not studying in their first choice of professional discipline reported that they would have chosen another health-related field, indicating that much of the homogeneity within speech-language pathology reflects the values and attributes of a wider social grouping.

Similarly, the predominance of females in the profession (91% to 98%) across a wide range of countries (Pickering et al., 1998) is not a feature of speech-language pathology alone, because for other related professions, particularly those working with young children such as in teaching, gender also is an issue (Cushman, 2005). A study of male speech-language pathology students and practitioners (McAllister & Neve, 2005) identified the tendency for males to come to the profession after experiencing another career path, frequently prompted by positive experiences with speech-language pathology services (for themselves or family member); this pattern of the influence of personal familiarity is shared by female prospective students in both speech-language pathology and other allied health professions (Byrne, 2005, 2006, 2007; Stewart et al., 2002). It may be that the powerful influence of personal familiarity conflates with the gender issues, so that young men (despite being more likely to directly experience speech-pathology services) may be less likely (owing to gender-related role expectations) to have other experiences with children and adults that provide indirect, profession-related familiarity. It is not uncommon for the numerical minority of males within the speech-language pathology profession to be regarded within a similar frame as that used in considering culturally oppressed minorities. Thus, McAllister & Neve (2005) describe female domination of the profession as a problem for males in terms of social isolation and potential for feeling overwhelmed, when in fact none of the males surveyed reported this as a problem; indeed, they reported high satisfaction as well as a consciousness of some advantages associated with being male (in line with wider social advantages of the male gender). From a feminist perspective, it is important to recognize that males experience no educational disadvantage before application for speech-language pathology programs that work against their entry, nor are selection procedures geared to discriminate on the basis of gender. From a critical perspective, it can be argued that the issues relate to widespread power inequity in the community with regard to expected gender roles. Historically, the profession was approximately 20% male in its early development in the 1930s, and possibly the reduction in the proportion of males in the profession reflects wider societal trends: Once the high-status early pioneering and technical developments have progressed sufficiently for tasks and roles to become routine, then status drops, as does the proportion of males. This phenomenon is evidenced in the early male dominance of secretarial roles, including those requiring shorthand and typing, at the turn of the twentieth century, compared with today. Although some argue that speech-language pathology would enhance its social power through being represented by more male professionals, this misses the important feminist argument signaled by Shapiro's (1994) discussion: Feminism aims to liberate men as much as women from cultural stereotyping, and rather than seeking men to "masculinize" speech-language pathology, speech-language pathology offers professionals of both genders the opportunity to make a difference by providing an important need in society.

As noted in Chapter 8, the discipline needs bilingual speech-language pathologists and also practitioners with learning experiences that promote the development of intercultural competence. Again, this is an international issue:

Cultural diversity is a feature of the general population across Australia, Canada, Hong Kong, South Africa, the United Kingdom, and the United States (Pickering et al., 1998). The primary factor of relevance here is recruitment strategies (Saenz, 2000; Stewart & Gonzalez, 2002; Stewart et al., 2002), because prior educational disadvantage can work against applicants for speech-language pathology programs even though selection procedures can appear neutral. Just as with the other issues of relevance here, lack of significant cultural and linguistic diversity is an issue of concern shared across allied health disciplines generally (Baldwin, Woods, & Simmons, 2006), and little has changed despite the fact that this is a long-standing issue. At one university, however, cultural and linguistic diversity was addressed explicitly by implementation of a project that successfully increased the multicultural learning opportunities in both academic and professional experience settings (Saenz, Wyatt, & Reinard, 1998). The change was effected by a shift in recruitment strategies that enabled consideration of multicultural experience, as well as academic and clinical potential (based on relevant work experience and referee reports), as well as entry on academic performance. The investigators reported that between 1992 and 1997, the proportion of minority undergraduates at their university went from 19% to 41%, and the proportion of minority graduate students went from 14% to 30%. One of the "big wins" of this strategy was that as more students from the diverse groups accrued, the social support for minority students increased, which, argued the investigators, assisted the students' learning. In this program, cultural and linguistic diversity was recognized as adding value, for example, to program graduates' ability to provide services to clients from multicultural backgrounds.

In Greenwood and colleagues' (2006) study in the United Kingdom (previously discussed), it was found that students from minority ethnic backgrounds were less likely to be aware of the profession, and to know that a degree was involved, and tended to see speech and language therapy as being of lower status in terms of extent of scientific basis, relative professional status, and salary. These investigators argue that more public awareness is needed to assist recruitment (to increase diversity in terms of culture and gender); accordingly, as suggested earlier, directing such public awareness–raising activities toward particular cultural groupings with the community would appear to be warranted.

Deconstructing the "Expert"

This book has focused on expert practice, so it is fitting to close with a critical examination of the notion of *expert*. Duchan argues that the professional association in the United States (the American Academy of Speech Correction) was set up with restrictive criteria for entry (in terms of experience, qualifications, ethical reputation, and publication record), with the aim of establishing credentials of the emerging profession, but also " . . . in doing so [the founders] created an elite role for themselves that excluded other less-

educated, unpublished practitioners in the field" (J. F. Duchan, 2004, p. 3). Currently, entry is restricted in accordance with a minimum level of expertise, rather than 'expert' practice. The professional association, however, locates expertise through different levels of membership and awards. Duchan argues that this historical bid for professional status through establishment of an elite group had significant consequences for practice—for example, driving the medical diagnostic category approach, rather than a functional approach, and the strong reliance on the scientific paradigm (still continued through evidence-based practice today, as discussed in Chapter 8). Duchan suggests that this stance drove a wedge between theory and practice and between practitioners and people with communication disorders: If the "workers" (p. 7) had been organizing the association, things might have been done differently. This discussion resonates strongly with a critical discourse perspective in that the experts in the profession, once powerful enough to gain social recognition (sufficient to form a recognized association), are able to create more power and to develop more exclusive knowledge to sustain their power.

From a critical discourse perspective, the notion of *expert* creates a binary opposition with *novice*, with the power of the "knower" invested in the expert. Such an opposition raises the issue of the social agenda achieved through such a power distinction. Part of this picture is the notion of professionalism, and the discourse that surrounds that notion is heavily positivist—that is, it is through the claim to science that speech-language pathologists have attained the societal status that enables autonomy of the profession to provide services and to deem what knowledge is to constitute the disciplinary base. From a postmodern perspective, such science is, as Skrtic (1995) says, a " . . . form of cultural engagement between an object of study and a community of observers who are conditioned by their paradigm to see the object in a particular way" (p. 15). Within this frame, expert status can be seen as that accorded to persons within that community who are most conservatively engaged within that particular paradigm. This conservative rigidity is consistent with one of the commonly discussed features associated with expert practice, that of pattern recognition and production as an indicator of the extent to which experts have automatized practice. The danger for experts, as discussed in the preface of this book, is that the more expertise is gained, the less able is the practitioner to "unpack" or deconstruct practice. Deconstruction as described by Derrida (2004) is not a negative thing, because the emphasis for Derrida was on the "construction" of meanings (Smith, 2005)—so the deconstruction of expert practice is an attempt to understand how practice is understood and constructed within the community of practice, and within the wider community. Through this process of unpacking, experts can check on what they are doing, and so can teach others, and most important, they too can continue developing. This idea of deliberate action to de- and re-construct practice links closely to the idea that expert practice, to the level of mastery, requires more than simply increasingly more practice, instead requiring deliberate action to fundamentally reshape

practice (Ericsson & Charness, 1997). In this book, it has been suggested that a critical discourse perspective provides important tools to problematize expert practice, in order to make this shift into mastery.

References

Adamson, B. J., Covic, T., Kench, P. L., & Lincoln, M. (2003). Determinants of undergraduate program choice in two health science fields: Does personality influence career choice? *Focus on Health Professional Education: A Multi-Disciplinary Journal, 5*(2), 34–47.

Baldwin, A., Woods, K., & Simmons, M. C. (2006). Diversity of the allied health workforce: The unmet challenge. *Journal of Allied Health, 35*(2), 116–120.

Bartlett, T. (2004). Mapping distinction: Towards a systemic representation of power in language. In L. Young & C. Harrison (Eds.), *Systemic functional linguistics and critical discourse analysis* (pp. 68–84). London: Continuum.

Butt, D., Fahey, R., Feez, S., Spinks, S., & Yallop, C. (2000). *Using functional grammar: An explorer's guide* (2nd ed.). Sydney: National Centre for English Language Teaching and Research.

Byrne, N. (2005). Career choice and speech pathology. *ACQuiring Knowledge in Speech, Language and Hearing, 7*(1), 16–18.

Byrne, N. (2006). *Therapy exposure to allied health and choosing that allied health profession as a career.* Paper presented at the ANZAME conference: Filling in the gaps, Gold Coast, Australia, June 29–July 2.

Byrne, N. (2007). *Factors influencing career choice in speech pathology*: Unpublished PhD thesis, University of Newcastle, Newcastle, Australia.

Carlson, M. (2004). A critical look at the construction of power between Applied Linguistic and Critical Applied Linguistics. *International Journal of Applied Linguistics, 14*(2), 167–184.

Chilton, P. (2005). Missing links in mainstream CDA: Modules, blends and the critical instinct. In R. Wodak & P. Chilton (Eds.), *A new agenda in (critical) discourse analysis: Theory, methodology and interdisciplinarity* (pp. 19–51). Amsterdam: John Benjamins.

Code, C., Simmons-Mackie, N., Armstrong, E., Stiegler, L., Armstrong, J., Bushby, E., et al. (2001). The public awareness of aphasia: An international survey. *International Journal of Language & Communication Disorders, 36*(Suppl.), 1–6.

Coulthard, M. (Ed.). (1992). *Advances in spoken discourse analysis.* London: Routledge.

Creswell, J. W. (2003). *Research design: Qualitative, quantitative and mixed method approaches.* Thousand Oaks, CA: Sage.

Cushman, P. (2005). It's just not a real bloke's job: Male teachers in the primary school. *Asia-Pacific Journal of Teacher Education, 33*(3), 321–338.

Daniels, D. E., & Gabel, R. M. (2004). The impact of stuttering on identity construction. *Topics in Language Disorders, 24*(3), 200–215.

de Beaugrande, R. (2001). Interpreting the discourse of H.G. Widdowson: A corpus-based critical discourse analysis. *Applied Linguistics, 22*(1), 104–121.

Deal, M. (2003). Disabled people's attitudes toward other impairment groups: A hierarchy of impairments. *Disability & Society, 18*(7), 897–910.

Derrida, J. (2004). *Positions* (A. Bass, Trans. Originally published in France in 1972 as Positions by Les Editions de Minuit ed.). London: Continuum.

Duchan, J. (2002, December). What do you know about the history of speech-language pathology? *ASHA Leader, 7,* 4–5, 29.

Duchan, J. F. (2004). *Professional identity: Then and now.* Retrieved Oct. 30, 2006, from www.speechpathology.com/articles/pf_article_detail.asp?article_id=69

Eadie, P. (2005). The case for public speech pathology terminology: Recognizing *Dianthus caryophyllus? Advances in Speech-Language Pathology, 7*(2), 91–93.

Eggins, S. (1994). *An introduction to systemic functional linguistics.* London: Pinter.

Eggins, S., & Slade, D. (2004). *Analysing casual conversation.* London/New York: Equinox/Cassell.

Eldridge, M. (1968). *A history of the treatment of speech disorders.* Edinburgh: E. & S. Livingstone Ltd.

Elman, R. J., Ogar, J., & Elman, S. H. (2000). Aphasia: Awareness, advocacy, and activism. *Aphasiology, 14*(5/6), 455–459.

Ericsson, K. A., & Charness, N. (1997). Cognitive and developmental factors in expert performance. In P. J. Feltovich, K. M. Ford, & R. R. Hoffman (Eds.), *Expertise in context: Human and machine* (pp. 3–41). Menlo Park, CA: AAAI Press/MIT Press.

Fairclough, N. (2004). Semiotic aspects of social transformation and learning. In R. Rogers (Ed.), *An introduction to critical discourse analysis in education* (pp. 225–235). Mahwah, NJ: Lawrence Erlbaum Associates.

Foucault, M. (2000). Interview with Michel Foucault (R. Hurley, Trans.). In J. D. Faubion (Ed.), *Power (Vol.3: Essential works of Foucault 1954–1984, ed. P. Rainbow)* (pp. 259–297). New York: The New Press.

Foucault, M. (2001). *Dits et ecrits (Vol. I: 1954–1975).* Paris, France: Gallimard.

Gaventa, J., & Cornwall, A. (2001). Power and knowledge. In P. Reason & H. Bradbury (Eds.), *Handbook of action research: Participative inquiry and practice* (pp. 70–80). London: Sage.

Goffman, E. (1968). *Stigma: Notes on the management of spoiled identity.* Harmondsworth, UK: Penguin.

Greenwood, N., Wright, J., & Bithell, C. (2006). Perceptions of speech and language therapy amongst UK school and college students: Implications for recruitment. *International Journal of Language & Communication Disorders, 41*(1), 83–94.

Hagstrom, F., & Wertsch, J. V. (2004). Grounding social identity for professional practice. *Topics in Language Disorders, 24*(3), 162–173.

Halliday, M. A. K., & Matthiessen, C. M. I. M. (2004). *An introduction to functional grammar* (3rd ed.). London: Arnold.

Hammersley, M. (2003). Conversation analysis and discourse analysis: Methods or paradigms? *Discourse & Society, 14*(6), 751–781.

Johnston, R. (2000). Whose side, whose research, whose learning, whose outcomes? Ethics, emancipatory research and unemployment. In H. Simons & R. Usher (Eds.), *Situated ethics in educational research* (pp. 69–81). London: Routledge-Falmer.

Kemmis, S. (2001). Exploring the relevance of critical theory for action research: Emancipatory action research in the footsteps of Jurgen Habermas. In P. Reason & H. Bradbury (Eds.), *Handbook of action research: Participative inquiry and practice* (pp. 91–102). London: Sage.

Killarney, G. T., & Lass, N. J. (1981, June). A survey of rural public awareness of speech-language pathology and audiology. *ASHA*, 415–419.

Klein, J. F., & Hood, S. B. (2004). The impact of stuttering on employment opportunities and job performance. *Journal of Fluency Disorders, 29*, 255–273.

Kress, G. (1990). Critical discourse analysis. *Annual Review of Applied Linguistics, 11*, 84–99.

Kuhn, T. S. (1970). *The structure of scientific revolutions* (2nd ed.). Chicago: University of Chicago Press.

Lesser, R., & Hassip, S. (1986). Knowledge and opinions of speech therapy in teachers, doctors and nurses. *Child: Care, Health & Development, 12*, 235–249.

Lupton, D. (1992). Discourse analysis: A new methodology for understanding the ideologies of health and illness. *Australian Journal of Public Health, 16*(2), 145–150.

Martin, J. R., Matthiessen, C. M. I. M., & Painter, C. (1997). *Working with functional grammar*. London: Arnold.

Martin, J. R., & Rose, D. (2003). *Working with discourse: Meaning beyond the clause*. London: Continuum.

Matthiessen, C. M. I. M., & Halliday, M. A. K. (1997). *Systemic functional grammar: A first step into the theory*. Sydney: Macquarie University.

McAllister, L., & Neve, B. (2005). Male students and practitioners in speech pathology: An Australian pilot study. In C. Heine & L. Brown (Eds.), *Proceedings of the 2005 Speech Pathology Australia national conference: Practicality and impact —making a difference in the real world* (pp. 127–134). Melbourne: Speech Pathology Australia.

Nordholm, L. A., & Westbrook, M. T. (1978). Students entering speech pathology and other health professions: Their backgrounds, attitudes and aspirations. *Australian Journal of Human Communication Disorders, 6*(1), 60–68.

Norris, S., & Jones, R. H. (Eds.). (2005). *Discourse in action: Introducing mediated discourse analysis*. London: Routledge.

O'Callaghan, A. M., McAllister, L., & Wilson, L. (2005). Barriers to accessing rural paediatric speech pathology services: Health care consumers' perspectives. *Australian Journal of Rural Health, 13*, 162–171.

O'Neill, Y. V. (1980). *Speech and speech disorders in Western thought before 1600*. Westport, Connecticut: Greenwood Press.

Parr, S., Byng, S., Gilpin, S., & Ireland, C. (1997). "They cannot see it so how will they know?": Aphasia and disability. In *Talking about aphasia* (pp. 117–133). Maidenhead, UK: Open University Press.

Parsons, C. L., Bowman, S. N., & Iacono, T. (1983). Public awareness of speech/language pathologists and the services they provide. *Australian Journal of Human Communication Disorders, 11*(1), 51–59.

Pennycook, A. (2001). *Critical applied linguistics: A critical introduction*. Mahwah, NJ: Lawrence Erlbaum Associates.

Pickering, M., McAllister, L., Hagler, P., Whitehill, T. L., Penn, C., Robertson, S. J., et al. (1998). External factors influencing the profession in six societies. *American Journal of Speech-Language Pathology, 7*(4), 5–17.

Preston, D. R. (1996). Whaddyaknow?: The modes of folk linguistic awareness. *Language Awareness, 5*(1), 40–74.

Prevignano, C. L., & Thibault, P. J. (Eds.). (2003). *Discussing conversation analysis.* Amsterdam: John Benjamins.

Reason, P., & Bradbury, H. (Eds.). (2001). *Handbook of action research: Participative inquiry and practice.* London: Sage.

Rowe, S. (2004). Discourse in activity and activity as discourse. In R. Rogers (Ed.), *An introduction to critical discourse analysis in education* (pp. 79–96). Mahwah, NJ: Lawrence Erlbaum Associates.

Saenz, T. I. (2000). Issues in recruitment and retention of graduate students. *Communication Disorders Quarterly, 21*(4), 246–250.

Saenz, T. I., Wyatt, T. A., & Reinard, J. C. (1998). Increasing the recruitment and retention of historically underrepresented minority students in higher education: A case study. *American Journal of Speech-Language Pathology, 7*(3), 39–48.

Salas-Provance, M. B., Erickson, J. G., & Reed, J. (2002). Disabilities as viewed by four generations of one Hispanic family. *American Journal of Speech-Language Pathology, 11*(2), 151–162.

Shapiro, D. A. (1994, November). Tender gender issues. *ASHA*, 46–49.

Simmons-Mackie, N., Code, C., Armstrong, E., Stiegler, L., & Elman, R. J. (2002). What is aphasia? Results of an international survey. *Aphasiology, 16*(8), 837–848.

Skrtic, T. M. (1995). Theory/practice and objectivism: The modern view of the professions. In T. M. Skrtic (Ed.), *Disability and democracy: Reconstructing (special) education for postmodernity* (pp. 3–23). New York: Teachers College Press.

Smith, J. (2005). *Jacques Derrida: Live theory.* New York: Continuum.

Stewart, S. R., & Gonzalez, L. S. (2002). Serving a diverse population: The role of speech-language pathology professional preparation programs. *Journal of Allied Health, 31*(4), 204–216.

Stewart, S. R., Pool, J. B., & Winn, J. (2002). Factors in recruitment and employment of allied health students: Preliminary findings. *Journal of Allied Health, 31*(2), 111–116.

Sullivan, A., & Cleave, P. L. (2003). Knowledge of the roles of speech-language pathologists by students in other health care programs. *Journal of Speech-Language Pathology & Audiology, 27*(2), 98–107.

Survey report on general public perceptions on speech pathology and its meaning. (1995). Canterbury,Victoria, Australia: IER Ltd (Strategy Planning Consultants).

Thompson, G. (1996). *Introducing functional grammar.* London: Arnold.

Thompson, J. B. (1984). *Studies in the theory of ideology.* Cambridge: Polity Press.

Van Dijk, T. A. (2006). Discourse, context and cognition. *Discourse Studies, 8*(1), 159–177.

Van Dijk, T. A., & Kintsch, W. (1983). *Strategies of discourse comprehension.* New York: Academic Press.

Widdowson, H. G. (2000). On the limitations of linguistics applied. *Applied Linguistics, 21*(1), 3–25.

Young, L., & Harrison, C. (Eds.). (2004). *Systemic functional linguistics and critical discourse analysis.* London: Continuum.

Index

triangulation, 30–32, 45, 49, 168
types of discourse (*see* genre)

U

university, 111, 142, 152, 153, 182

V

validity of assessment, 13, 14, 16, 19–24,
    26, 29, 31, 36, 38, 51, 117, 132, 171
virtual, 119, 150
Visual Analogue Self-Esteem Scale, 37
voice
    disorder, 14, 176, 180
    of the patient/client/learner, 62–64,
        98, 121, 141, 172
Vygotsky, 116, 121, 167

W

Washback, 36
Wenger, 11, 116
Western Aphasia Battery, 25, 48, 80
workplace, 48, 54, 91, 97, 98, 110, 111,
    116–122, 127, 130, 131, 133, 134,
    139, 147, 148, 157, 158
World Health Organization (WHO)
    framework, 7
writing
    assessment of, 46, 99, 118–120
    reports, 47, 95–98

Z

zone of proximal development, 128